Techniques in Facial Plastic Surgery: Discussion and Debate part 2

Editors

FRED G. FEDOK
ROBERT M. KELLMAN

FACIAL PLASTIC SURGERY CLINICS OF NORTH AMERICA

www.facialplastic.theclinics.com

Consulting Editor
J. REGAN THOMAS

February 2014 • Volume 22 • Number 1

ELSEVIER

1600 John F. Kennedy Boulevard • Suite 1800 • Philadelphia, Pennsylvania, 19103-2899

http://www.theclinics.com

FACIAL PLASTIC SURGERY CLINICS OF NORTH AMERICA Volume 22, Number 1
February 2014 ISSN 1064-7406, ISBN-13: 978-1-4557-3860-1

Editor: Joanne Husovski

Facial Plastic Surgery Clinics of North America (ISSN 1064-7406) is published quarterly by Elsevier Inc., 360 Park Avenue South, New York, NY 10010-1710. Months of issue are February, May, August, and November. Business and Editorial Offices: 1600 John F. Kennedy Blvd., Suite 1800, Philadelphia, PA 19103-2899. Periodicals postage paid at New York, NY, and additional mailing offices. Subscription prices are $390.00 per year (US individuals), $525.00 per year (US institutions), $445.00 per year (Canadian individuals), $653.00 per year (Canadian institutions), $535.00 per year (foreign individuals), $653.00 per year (foreign institutions), $185.00 per year (US students), and $255.00 per year (foreign students). Foreign air speed delivery is included in all *Clinics* subscription prices. All prices are subject to change without notice. POSTMASTER: Send address changes to *Facial Plastic Surgery Clinics*, Elsevier Health Sciences Division, Subscription Customer Service, 3251 Riverport Lane, Maryland Heights, MO 63043. **Customer service: 1-800-654-2452 (US and Canada); 1-314-447-8871 (outside US and Canada); Fax: 314-447-8029; E-mail:journalscustomerservice-usa@elsevier.com (for print support); journalsonline support-usa@elsevier.com (for online support).**

Reprints. For copies of 100 or more of articles in this publication, please contact the Commercial Reprints Department, Elsevier Inc., 360 Park Avenue South, New York, NY 10010-1710. Tel.: 212-633-3874; Fax: 212-633-3820; E-mail: reprints@elsevier.com.

Facial Plastic Surgery Clinics of North America is covered in *MEDLINE/PubMed* (*Index Medicus*).

Printed and bound by CPI Group (UK) Ltd, Croydon, CR0 4YY

Transferred to digital print 2012

Contributors

CONSULTING EDITOR

J. REGAN THOMAS, MD, FACS
Professor and Chairman, Department of
Otolaryngology, University of Illinois at
Chicago, Chicago, Illinois

EDITORS

ROBERT M. KELLMAN, MD
Professor and Chair, Department of
Otolaryngology and Communication Sciences,
State University of New York–Upstate Medical
University, Syracuse, New York

FRED G. FEDOK, MD
Professor, Facial Plastic and Reconstructive
Surgery, Otolaryngology/Head and Neck
Surgery, Department of Surgery, The Hershey
Medical Center, The Pennsylvania State
University, Hershey, Pennsylvania

AUTHORS

PETER A. ADAMSON, MD, FRCSC, FACS
Professor and Head, Division of Facial Plastic
and Reconstructive Surgery Department of
Otolaryngology - Head and Neck Surgery,
University Health Network, University of
Toronto; Adamson Cosmetic Facial Surgery,
Toronto, Ontario, Canada

MARCELO B. ANTUNES, MD
Antunes Center for Facial Plastic Surgery,
Austin, Texas

SHAN BAKER, MD
Professor, Facial Plastic and Reconstructive
Surgery, Department of Otolayngology, Head
and Neck Surgery, University of Michigan,
Ann Arbor, Michigan

DANIEL BECKER, MD
Becker Nose and Sinus Center, Sewell, New
Jersey; Clinical Professor, Division of Facial
Plastic and Reconstructive Surgery,
Department of Otolaryngology, University of
Pennsylvania, Philadelphia, Pennsylvania

MINAS CONSTANTINIDES, MD
Assistant Professor, Department of
Otolaryngology, New York University School of

Medicine & New York Head & Neck Institute,
New York, New York

EDWIN ALAN CORTEZ, MD, FACS
Cortez Facial Plastic Surgery, Overland Park,
Kansas

FRED G. FEDOK, MD, FACS
Professor and Chief, Facial Plastic and
Reconstructive Surgery, Division of
Otolaryngology/Head and Neck Surgery,
Department of Surgery, The Hershey Medical
Center, Pennsylvania State University,
Hershey, Pennsylvania

GREG KELLER, MD
Keller Facial Plastic Surgery, David Geffen
School of Medicine, University of California,
Los Angeles, Santa Barbara, California

ALYN J. KIM, MD
University of Toronto; Adamson Cosmetic
Facial Surgery, Toronto, Ontario, Canada

KEITH LAFERRIERE, MD
Mercy Clinic - Facial Plastic Surgery,
Springfield, Missouri

WAYNE F. LARRABEE Jr, MD
Director, Larrabee Center for Facial Plastic Surgery; Clinical Professor, Department of Otolaryngology, Head and Neck Surgery, University of Washington, Seattle, Washington

CHRISTINA K. MAGILL, MD
Division of Facial Plastic and Reconstructive Surgery, Department of Otolaryngology - Head and Neck Surgery, University of California-Davis, Sacramento, California

DEVINDER S. MANGAT, MD
Clinical Professor for Facial Plastic Surgery, Department of Otolaryngology/Head and Neck Surgery, Mangat-Kuy-Holzpfel Plastic Surgery, University of Cincinnati; Private Practice, Cincinnati, Ohio; Private Practice, Vail, Colorado

STEVEN PEARLMAN, MD
Associate Clinical Professor, Columbia University, New York, New York; Director, Center for Aesthetic Facial Surgery, New York Head and Neck Institute, Manhattan Eye Ear and Throat Hospital, Lenox Hill Hospital, Northshore-L I J Hospital System, New York, New York

VITO C. QUATELA, MD
Quatela Center for Plastic Surgery, Rochester, New York

THOMAS J. ROMO III, MD, FACS
The Manhattan Eye, Ear and Throat Hospital, Director of Facial Plastic and Reconstructive Surgery, Lenox Hill Hospital, New York, New York

RAHUL SETH, MD
Assistant Professor, Department of Otolaryngology- Head and Neck Surgery, Division of Facial Plastic and Reconstructive Surgery, University of California, San Francisco, San Francisco, California

JAMES SIDMAN, MD
Director, ENT and Facial Plastic Surgery, Children's Hospitals and Clinics of Minnesota, University of Minnesota Medical School, Minneapolis, Minnesota

JONATHAN M. SYKES, MD
Professor and Director, Facial Plastic Surgery, University of California-Davis Medical Center, Sacramento, California

SHERARD AUSTIN TATUM, MD, FAAP, FACS
Professor of Otolaryngology and Pediatrics, Upstate Medical University, State University of New York, Syracuse, New York

DEAN M. TORIUMI, MD
Professor, Division of Facial Plastic and Reconstructive Surgery, Department of Otolaryngology - Head & Neck Surgery, University of Illinois at Chicago, Chicago, Illinois

JEREMY WARNER, MD, FACS
Assistant Clinical Professor, Division of Facial Plastic Surgery, University of Chicago, Chicago, Illinois; NorthShore University Health System, Director of Facial Plastic Surgery, Northbrook, Illinois

Contents

FACIAL PLASTIC SURGERY CLINICS OF NORTH AMERICA

FORTHCOMING ISSUES

Neck Rejuvenation: Surgical and Non-Surgical
Mark M. Hamilton, MD and Mark M. Beaty, MD, *Editors*

Facial Plastic Surgery Multicultural Aesthetics
J. Regan Thomas, MD, *Editor*

Pediatric Facial Reconstruction
Sherard S. Tatum MD, *Editor*

RECENT ISSUES

November 2013
Complications in Facial Plastic Surgery
Richard L. Goode, MD and Sam P. Most, *Editors*

August 2013
Hair Restoration
Raymond J. Konior, MD, FACS and
Steven P. Gabel, MD, FACS, *Editors*

May 2013
Minimally Invasive Procedures in Facial Plastic Surgery
Theda C. Kontis, *Editor*

RELATED INTEREST

Clinics in Plastic Surgery, Volume 40, Issue 2, April 2013
Outcomes Measures in Plastic Surgery
Kevin C. Chung, MD, MS and Andrea L. Pusic, MD, MHS, *Editors*

Advisory Board to Facial Plastic Surgery Clinics 2014

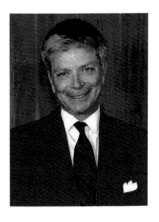
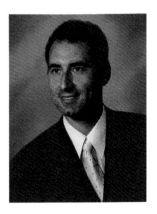
Facial Plastic Surgery Clinics is pleased to introduce the 2014-2015 **Advisory Board**.

Facial Plastic Surgery Clinics is widely available through the media of print, digital e-Reader, online via the Internet, and on iPad and smart phones.

Facial Plastic Surgery Clinics provides professionals access to pertinent point-of-care answers and current clinical information, along with comprehensive background information for deeper understanding.

Readers are welcome to contact the Clinics Editor or Board with comments.

BOARD MEMBERS 2014

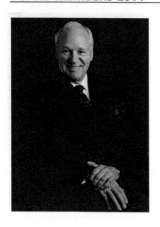

PETER A. ADAMSON, MD

Professor and Head
Division of Facial Plastic and Reconstructive Surgery
Department of Otolaryngology–Head and Neck Surgery
University of Toronto
Toronto, Ontario, Canada

Adamson Cosmetic Facial Surgery
Renaissance Plaza; 150 Bloor Street West; Suite M110
Toronto, Ontario M5S 2X9

416.323.3900
paa@dradamson.com
www.dradamson.com

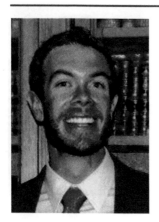

BENJAMIN P. CAUGHLIN, MD

Department of Otolaryngology
1855 W. Taylor Room 2.42
Chicago, IL 60612

312.996.1545
benjamincaughlin@gmail.com

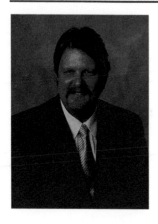

RICK DAVIS, MD

Voluntary Professor
The University of Miami Miller School of Medicine
Miami, Florida

The Center for Facial Restoration
1951 S.W. 172nd Ave; Suite 205
Miramar, Florida 33029

954.442.5191
drd@davisrhinoplasty.com
www.DavisRhinoplasty.com

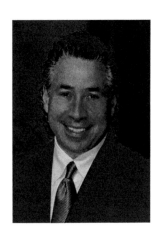
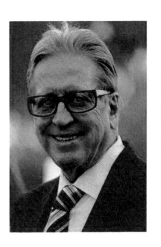
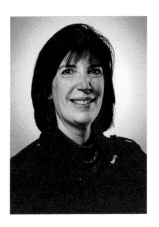

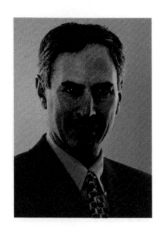

IRA D. PAPEL, MD

Facial Plastic Surgicenter
Associate Professor
The Johns Hopkins University
1838 Greene Tree Road, Suite 370
Baltimore, MD 21208

410.486.3400
idpmd@aol.com
www.facial-plasticsurgery.com

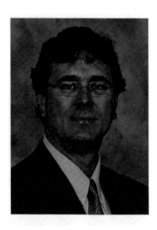

SHERARD A. TATUM, MD

Professor of Otolaryngology and
Pediatrics Cleft and Craniofacial Center
Division of Facial Plastic Surgery
Upstate Medical University
750 E. Adams St.
Syracuse, NY 13210

315.464.4636
TatumS@upstate.edu
www.upstate.edu

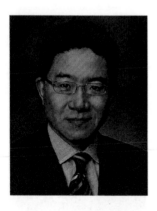

TOM D. WANG, MD

Professor
Facial Plastic and Reconstructive Surgery
Oregon Health & Science University
3181 Southwest Sam Jackson Park Road
Portland, OR 97239

503.494.5678
wangt@ohsu.edu
www.ohsu.edu/drtomwang

Preface

Discussion and Debate Among Facial Plastic Surgeons: Everyone Wins

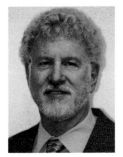 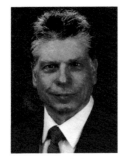

Robert M. Kellman, MD   Fred G. Fedok, MD

Editors

This is the second part of our discussion-and-debate issue that the publishers of *Facial Plastic Surgery Clinics of North America* were kind enough to allow us to develop. We started this concept of discussion and debate in print form based on a fairly simple concept. We set out to discover what were among the most compelling questions active practitioners of facial plastic surgery have in the selected areas. The goal was simple—in these areas of varied opinion, what were the most credible persons' thoughts in the topic area on selected questions. The questions were developed after inquiries with numerous facial plastic surgeons. The article panels were selected by invitation based on the authors' activity and publishing, research, and clinical practice. The questions were then posed to them in a manner that allowed independent thought, and a later opportunity to addend their answers, but not to change their initial impressions.

The first installment in the series was exceedingly successful. We humbly submit that the goals were achieved, and the readers were satisfied and gained insight into the practical opinions of their respected colleagues.

What this series does is allows an effective simulation of what is frequently the most sought after and popular aspect of a live meeting—the panel discussion.

Although the term debate usually implies a goal to achieve a "win" for a single participant, in this discussion and debate series the goal is really for all the participants and the readers to win. And through this interchange of knowledge our patients win! In this series the readers are allowed to "listen" to the opinions of the authors, to sample and weigh the assumptions of the authors, and to draw their own conclusions based on the varied opinions presented on each topic.

So once again we encourage you to read these sections with enthusiasm, with interest, and with intensity. Your own opinion based on what is written here becomes part of the working knowledge of facial plastic surgery. It is both a pleasure and a privilege to present to you this second series.

We give our highest praise and appreciation to Joanne Husovski, who has endured the corralling of not only your two editors here, but also a large number of authors. She executed the task

Facial Plast Surg Clin N Am 22 (2014) xiii–xiv
http://dx.doi.org/10.1016/j.fsc.2013.11.001
1064-7406/14/$ – see front matter © 2014 Elsevier Inc. All rights reserved.

well and here we present our next excellent installment.

Cordially,

Fred Fedok, Bob Kellman, and the publishers

Robert M. Kellman, MD
Department of Otolaryngology and
Communication Sciences
State University of New York–
Upstate Medical University
750 East Adams Street
Syracuse, NY 13210, USA

Fred G. Fedok, MD
Facial Plastic and Reconstructive Surgery
Otolaryngology/Head and Neck Surgery
Department of Surgery
The Hershey Medical Center
The Pennsylvania State University
500 University Drive
Hershey, PA 17033, USA

E-mail addresses:
kellmanr@upstate.edu (R.M. Kellman)
ffedok@hmc.psu.edu (F.G. Fedok)

Chemical Peels: Panel Discussion

Edwin Alan Cortez, MD[a,*], Fred G. Fedok, MD[b,*],
Devinder S. Mangat, MD[c,d,e,*]

KEYWORDS

- Chemical peels • Croton oil–phenol peel • Trichloroacetic acid • Jessner solution

---

Chemical Peels Panel Discussion

Edwin Cortez, Fred Fedok, and Devinder Mangat address questions for discussion and debate:

1. Do you agree or disagree, and why, with the following: "The best method to improve moderate to deep rhytids is the croton oil–phenol peel."

2. Do you agree or disagree, and why, with the following: "There are no problems with cardiotoxicity with croton oil–phenol peels if done appropriately."

3. Do you agree or disagree, and why, with the following: "Do not do spot testing with chemical peel agents."

4. How do you handle peels in advanced Fitzpatrick skin types III, IV, V?

5. What is the main factor for rate of reepithelialization: (1) depth of peel, (2) depth of laser, (3) depth of dermabrasion?

6. Analysis: How has your approach to or technique in chemical peels evolved over the past several years?

Two videos presented with this discussion accompany this article at http://www.facialplastic.
theclinics.com/. One is a demonstration of the technique of applying the croton oil peel by
Dr Edwin Cortez. The other is a 4-minute video showing short clips of Dr Fred Fedok performing a
35% TCA/Jessner peel and a Baker-Gordon peel, and clips showing the performance of using the
35% TCA/Jessner peel on one section of a patient's face and the Baker-Gordon Peel on another

Do you agree or disagree, and why, with the following: "the best method to improve moderate to deep rhytids is the croton oil–phenol peel."

CORTEZ

I fully agree with the statement that "the best method to improve moderate to deep rhytids is the croton oil–phenol peel (Video 1)." Phenol–croton oil peeling is still the standard against which all other treatment regimens for photodamaged skin are measured. In my practice, this modality is still the most safe, cost-efficient, and long-term treatment for treating medium and coarse facial rhytids. **Figs. 1** and **2** show 2 of our patients before and after treatment.

---

[a] Cortez Facial Plastic Surgery, 14241 Metcalf Avenue, Overland Park, KS 66223, USA; [b] Facial Plastic and Reconstructive Surgery, Division of Otolaryngology / Head and Neck Surgery, Department of Surgery, The Hershey Medical Center, Pennsylvania State University, 400 University Drive, Hershey, PA 17033, USA; [c] Department of Otolaryngology/Head and Neck Surgery, University of Cincinnati, 231 Albert Sabin Way, Cincinnati, OH 45267-0528, USA; [d] Private Practice, Mangat-Kuy-Holzapfel Plastic Surgery, 8044 Montgomery Rd - Suite 230, Cincinnati, OH 45236, USA; [e] Private Practice, Mangat Plastic Surgery Center, 0056 Edwards Village Boulevard - Suite 226, Edwards, CO 81632, USA
* Corresponding authors.
E-mail addresses: info@cortezfacialplasticsurgery.com (Cortez); drfredfedok@me.com (Fedok); mangat@fuse.net (Mangat)

Facial Plast Surg Clin N Am 22 (2014) 1–23
http://dx.doi.org/10.1016/j.fsc.2013.09.004

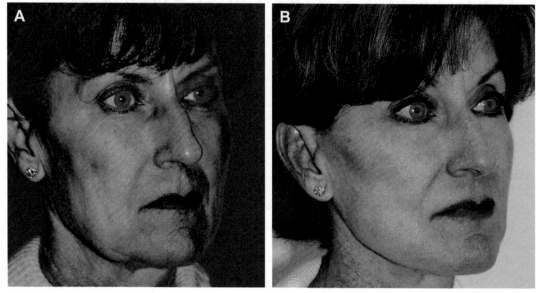

Fig. 1. Cortez. (A) Before croton oil–phenol peel. (B) Two years after croton oil–phenol peel.

The long-term criticisms of the standard Baker-Gordon peel are no longer valid. Since the elegant studies by Hetter and Stone, the entire spectrum of croton oil–phenol peeling has finally become scientifically validated. For many years, we were very pleased with our results from the Baker-Gordon formula but we have now created our own modification, which will be discussed in response to a different discussion. We have observed patients for over 25 years after being treated with croton oil–phenol preparations, and the long-term results are excellent. We are now seeing patients who we treated in their 50s and are now in their 70s and still have beautiful, firm,

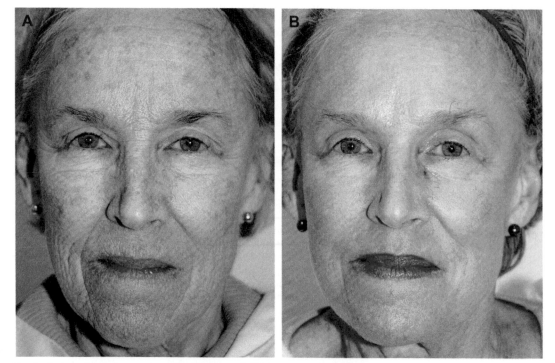

Fig. 2. Cortez. (A) Before croton oil–phenol peel. (B) One year after croton oil–phenol peel.

non-photodamaged skin. I have used dermabrasion for rhytids in the past, but in this day of problems with infectious diseases, including human immunodeficiency virus, hepatitis C, and so forth, I would prefer not to have aerosolization in my operating suite.

In the early 1990s we saw a dramatic shift to laser ablative resurfacing with the CO_2 laser. This modality was supposed to be free of any serious postoperative sequelae, such as hypopigmentation. However, 2 years after large numbers of cases were performed with the CO_2 laser, many patients were seen who developed severe hypopigmentation and also scarring and texture changes, and so forth. Now, many have put their CO_2 lasers in the garage and a new era of fractional CO_2 laser resurfacing has been born. We all hope that this expensive laser lives up to industries' promises!

In summary, to date, we still find the croton oil–phenol peel as the best and safest modality for the treatment of moderate and deep rhytids.

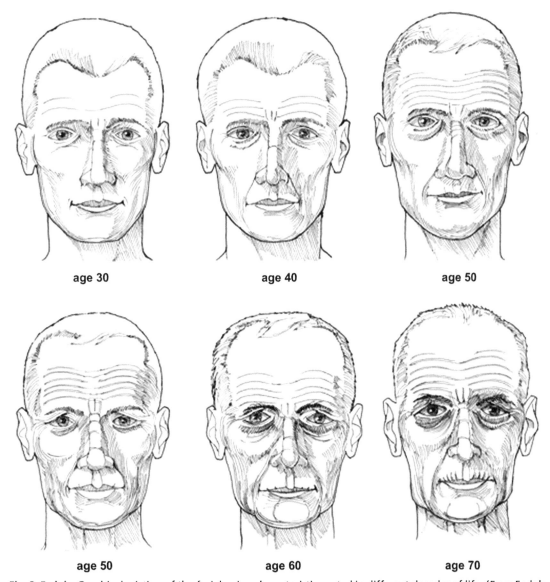

age 30   age 40   age 50

age 50   age 60   age 70

Fig. 3. Fedok. Graphic depiction of the facial aging characteristics noted in different decades of life. (*From* Fedok FG. Minimally invasive and office-based procedures in facial plastic surgery. New York: Thieme; 2014; with permission.)

FEDOK

The term "rhytids" describes the wrinkled appearance of the skin caused by the decrease in skin elasticity, decrease in skin water content, and changes in collagen crosslinking that typically occurs with aging.[1–6] In patients with milder aging effects, the rhytids are fairly superficial and the derangement of the anatomy is isolated to more superficial aspects of the epidermis and dermis, such as might be present in the facial skin of patients in their third decade. With more advanced skin aging the involutional and photoaging changes are more pronounced and involve deeper aspects of the dermis. In the former situation, such as in the younger patient, the rhytids usually make their early appearance around the "crow-feet" area and are largely noticeable with movement, such as smiling. In the latter situation more typical of the older patient, the rhytids may be present at repose and actually produce folds of lax skin with movement (**Fig. 3**).

Both these situations are manageable through a plethora of resurfacing techniques. The patient with milder aging skin is managed with a variety of less aggressive techniques and modalities. The latter situation of the patient with deeper rhytids is best managed by a combination of techniques including deeper resurfacing, surgery, and possibly the utilization of injected filling material. The extent of improvement of facial skin texture and rhytids can be anticipated depending on the resurfacing technique utilized.

Box 1[7] displays a classification system for the grading of the severity of photoaging. Deeper rhytids along with a number of other unfavorable skin characteristics are typically encountered in patients with Grade III and IV photoaging. These patients frequently present with rhytids at rest and with readily apparent folds and laxity. These unfavorable skin characteristics are secondary to severe full-thickness skin aging. The improvement of these deep rhytids is dependent on a

technique's ability to cause changes in the deeper portions of the skin.

The deeper peels with formulations based on phenol and croton oil are popularly represented as one of the standards against which all other resurfacing techniques can be compared. In my practice we have used the Baker-Gordon formulation for patients with deeper rhytids. When properly utilized in the appropriate candidate, this phenol-based peel achieves predictable and reproducibly favorable changes in skin texture and rhytids compared to other techniques. There is a wide safety margin when this peel is used by experienced practitioners. This favorable effect is only approximated by full ablative CO_2 resurfacing. In my experience, however, the Baker-Gordon formula chemical peel has produced the most remarkable results in appropriate patients with deeper rhytids, with a minimal occurrence of hyperpigmentation, spotty hypopigmentation, or other problems.[8–10]

> **Box 1**
> **Fedok. Patient selection: Glogau photoaging classification**
>
> - I. Mild (28–35 years)
>   - No keratosis, little wrinkling, no scarring, little or no makeup
> - II. Moderate (35–50 years)
>   - Early actinic and wrinkling, parallel smile lines, mild scarring, little makeup
> - III. Advanced (50–65 years)
>   - Actinic keratosis, telangiectasia, wrinkling, present at rest, always wears makeup
> - IV. Severe (60–75 years)
>   - Actinic keratosis, skin cancers, wrinkling, skin laxity, makeup does not cover, "cakes on"

MANGAT

The Baker-Gordon phenol-based peel was the gold standard for over 30 years for treating moderate to deep wrinkling on the face. This chemical peel, which was a single-strength peel, was all that was available for all skin types and various degrees of actinic damage other than the lighter and less effective trichloroacetic acid (TCA)-based peels. Between 1989 and 1995, Gregory Hetter MD carried out some groundbreaking clinical research regarding the efficacy and

legitimacy of the Baker-Gordon phenol/croton oil formula and proved that it is croton oil and not phenol that is the active ingredient in the "phenol" Baker-Gordon formula. Out of this research, Dr. Hetter came up with varying strengths of chemical peels based on the concentration of croton oil from 0.1% to 1.6% that consequently varies the depth of the peel and the effectiveness of treating actinic damage and, in particular, rhytids.

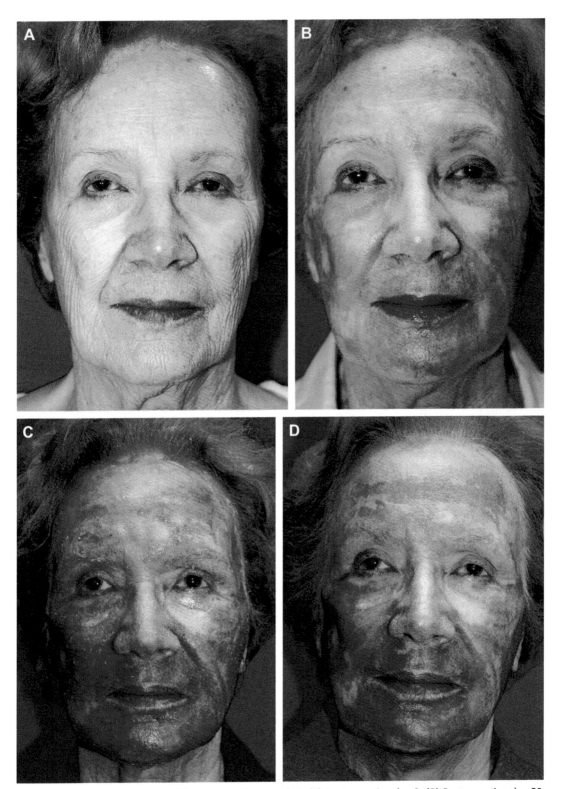

Fig. 4. Mangat. (*A*) Preoperative. (*B*) Postoperative month 3. (*C*) Postoperative day 8. (*D*) Postoperative day 20.

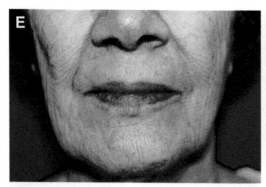
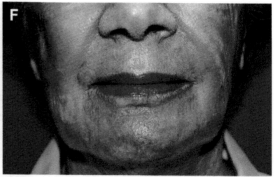

Fig. 4. Mangat. *(continued)* *(E)* Preoperative view of perioral area. *(F)* Perioral area 3 months postoperatively.

I would wholeheartedly agree that the best method to improve moderate to deep rhytids is the Hetter formulation of the croton oil–phenol peel, understanding that croton oil is the active ingredient rather than phenol. The varying strength of the chemical peel solution allows one to peel different areas of the face with the appropriate strength of solution based on the thickness of the skin and the extent of rhytids in each respective area. It is no longer necessary to use one-strength chemical peel solution for the entire face. As an example, one could use a 0.4% Hetter peel for the periorbital area, which has thinner skin with mild to moderate rhytids; 0.8% or 1.2% Hetter peel for the perioral area, which has thicker skin and deeper rhytids; and 0.2% Hetter solution for the cheeks, which may demonstrate only dyschromia and no rhytids. For areas that have simply lentigines and dyschromia, one could even use a USP 89% phenol solution with no croton oil and get very effective improvement with rapid reepithelialization and minimal postpeel erythema.

In my experience of performing chemical peels for 30 years and having performed CO_2 laser resurfacing for approximately 5 years, there was no doubt about the superiority of the chemical peel resurfacing technique over the CO_2 laser resurfacing modality, purely from the standpoint of eliminating rhytids and observing the extent of improvement in actinic damage, particularly in Fitzpatrick skin types I and II. That continues to be the case with newer Hetter peel formulations. The advantage now is that one can vary the

strength of the chemical peel on different parts of the face, thus reducing healing time, the extent of erythema post peel, and overall morbidity without sacrificing the result. As with the Baker-Gordon peel, the Hetter peel also demonstrates significant postpeel increase and reorganization of collagen in skin.

One of the biggest disadvantages of a resurfacing procedure, whether it is the use of a laser or the Baker-Gordon peel, is the extent of erythema seen in the postresurfacing period and the length of time to see a reduction/resolution of the redness.

With the Hetter formula and varying the strength of the peel formula used, the amount of erythema observed is significantly diminished and, consequently, the amount of time it takes for the erythema to resolve is likewise reduced to a significant degree. Furthermore, with the Hetter croton peel, the incidence of hypopigmentation has been virtually eliminated, particularly in the Fitzpatrick type I and II skin. In the past 10 years of performing the Hetter peel, I have observed no scarring or deep pigmentation of the skin as long as the patients are carefully selected. Utilizing the 0.1% or the 0.2% croton oil peel, one can easily treat actinic damage in the neck as well as the upper chest in a controlled manner to treat lentigines and dyschromia, with little or no risk of postpeel hypopigmentation or scarring. Until the advent of the Hetter croton oil peel, peeling the neck was extremely risky using any other peeling agents such as TCA or phenol.

See **Figs. 4–6** for Dr Mangat's clinical outcomes with the Hetter croton oil peel.

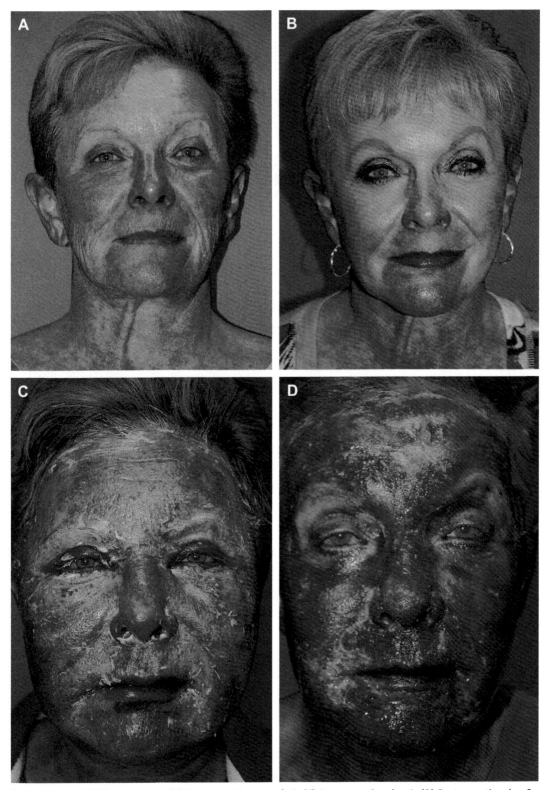

Fig. 5. Mangat. (*A*) Preoperative. (*B*) Postoperative month 7. (*C*) Postoperative day 1. (*D*) Postoperative day 6.

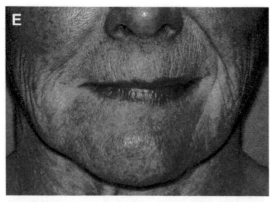 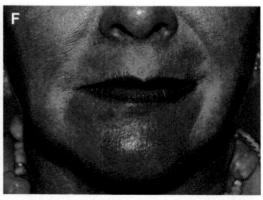

Fig. 5. Mangat. *(continued)* (*E*) Preoperative view of perioral area. (*F*) Perioral area 7 months postoperatively.

Do you agree or disagree, and why, with the following: "there are no problems with cardiotoxicity with croton oil–phenol peels if done appropriately."

CORTEZ

I completely agree that there are no problems with cardiotoxicity as long as the procedure is done appropriately. In personally performing over 1500 croton oil–phenol based peels, I have never seen any cardiac abnormality with full cardiac monitoring.

Historically, it has been taught that phenol and phenol-based formulas are cardiotoxic. Phenol has been shown to be directly toxic to the myocardium. In patients peeled rapidly, 50% of total surface in 30 minutes or less, tachycardia was noted initially, followed by premature ventricular contractions, premature atrial contractions, bigeminy, trigeminy, atrial tachycardia, and ventricular tachycardia. In contrast, when phenol was applied to 50% of the facial skin surface over 60 minutes, arrhythmias were not observed.

Thus, it appears that higher levels of phenol absorption produce myocardial irritability.

To avoid cardiotoxicity when performing croton oil–phenol peels, follow the following regimen:

1. Screen patients for cardiac disease.
2. Have appropriate cardiac monitoring before, during, and after the procedure.
3. Hydrate the patient before, during, and after the peel.
4. Peel in aesthetic units, usually 5 units with a time lapse of 10 to 15 minutes between units. The total time for the peel should be 60 to 90 minutes.

Following this regimen should allow you to avoid any cardiotoxicity when performing croton oil–phenol peel.

FEDOK

There are reported instances and concerns about the cardiotoxicity of croton oil–phenol based peels.[11–17] In contrast, since I entered cosmetic practice in 1991 I have not had a patient experience any significant ectopy or arrhythmia while undergoing a phenol-based chemical peel.

Nevertheless, prevention and precaution is advised. The following is recommended and is consistent with my practice:

- Perform full-face phenol-based peels with the patient under cardiac monitoring.
- Keep the patient well hydrated.
- Provide intravenous access.
- Avoid an excess of epinephrine in local anesthetics.
- A full-face chemical peel is carried out in a sequence approximating the major aesthetic units of the face, so for instance, the

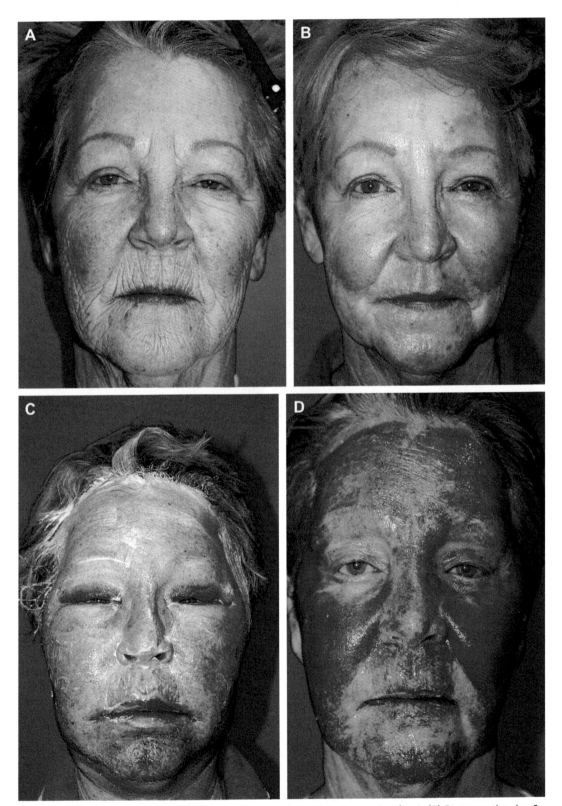

Fig. 6. Mangat. (*A*) Preoperative. (*B*) Postoperative month 6. (*C*) Postoperative day 1. (*D*) Postoperative day 6.

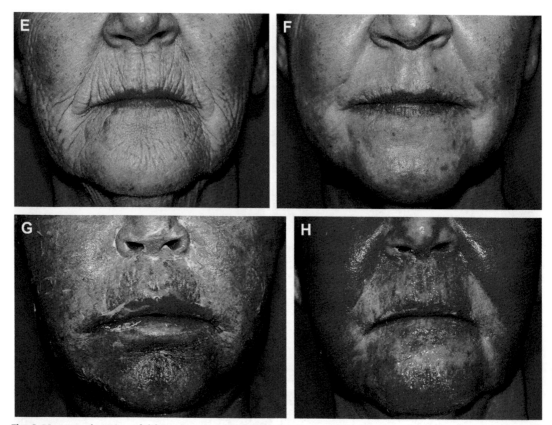

Fig. 6. Mangat. (*continued*) (*E*) Preoperative view of perioral area. (*F*) Perioral area 6 months postoperatively. (*G*) Perioral area on postoperative day 1. (*H*) Perioral area on postoperative day 6.

forehead is peeled first, then the periorbital areas, then the cheeks, and so forth, until the entire face is treated. There should be a several minute pause between each area, and the entire face should take approximately 75 to 90 minutes to be treated.

The rationale of the prolonged length of time between segments is to let any absorbed phenol to dilute and dissipate between treated sections to avoid creating an excessive serum level of phenol and resultant ectopy.

MANGAT

I would wholeheartedly agree that there are no problems with cardiotoxicity with any of the phenol or croton oil based chemical peels *if certain precautions are taken*. Cardiotoxicity is directly related to absorption of the phenol because high enough concentrations of phenol in the systemic circulation can cause ventricular extrasystoles and other arrhythmias. The same is certainly not the case with croton oil in any concentration. When we, formerly, performed the Baker-Gordon chemical peel, the following precautions were always taken:

1. Adequate prepeel intravenous hydration of the patient
2. Performing the peel in individual esthetic units, waiting at least 15 minutes between each unit, so that the full-face peel was performed over the course of 60 to 90 minutes
3. Preoperative, intraoperative, and postoperative ECG monitoring of every patient
4. Continue postoperatively intravenous hydration

Since the concentration of phenol in every Hetter solution is a constant 35%, the risk of cardiotoxicity with the Hetter peel is virtually nonexistent, allowing the operator to perform a full-face combination Hetter peel in a much shorter time period of no more than 30 minutes. The relative lack of cardiotoxicity with the Hetter–croton oil peel gives it an added advantage over the old Baker-Gordon peel.

Do you agree or disagree, and why, with the following: "do not do spot testing with chemical peel agents."

CORTEZ

I have treated several patients who have had spot testing with both phenol and TCA. These patients required full-face chemical peels to camouflage the test spot areas.

The rationale for performing spot testing with chemical peeling agents is both historical and anecdotal. The spot-testing concept came about because physicians thought that their patients and themselves would feel more secure if spot testing did not result in scarring or pigmentation abnormalities.

Frequently, these test spots were placed in the preauricular areas or just at the anterior hairline. These sites were selected because they could be covered with hair if the outcome was less than satisfactory. This scenario was not good if the patients decided not to proceed with the peel procedure because these patients had permanent relatively hypopigmented areas. Also, spot testing in 1 or 2 areas does not guarantee how the rest of the facial skin will respond. I have actually seen several patients who had croton oil–phenol test spots in the middle of each cheek with corresponding relative hypopigmentation. Of course, these patients required full-face peeling to create a desirable result. Somehow, the concept of easily camouflaged test spots was transformed into very observable areas, such as the mid and lateral cheeks.

In conclusion, I see the use of test spotting in chemical peel patients as an absolute contradiction. Physicians need to evaluate patients for chemical peeling by using history, physical exam, Fitzpatrick and Glogau classifications, and common sense.

FEDOK

In general I do not do spot testing with chemical peeling agents. Rarely, in isolated situations such as patients with Fitzpatrick III and Fitzpatrick IV skin types, especially when they have given a history or related other suspicion that they may have a tendency to hyperpigment, have I done this. In these cases I have done several small areas each proximally 1 to 2 cm^2 in size, peeling just adjacent to the hairline or in the postauricular area so that the area could be well camouflaged. Incidentally, in doing this I have not had an issue with unsightly hyperpigmentation or hypopigmentation.

MANGAT

I would disagree with this statement because in some situations and in some patients spot testing can be invaluable to avoid undesirable outcomes, although we agree that the croton oil–phenol peels should ideally be performed in patients with Fitzpatrick type I or type II skin.

The lower concentration croton oil peels as formulated by Hetter can be used for skin types III and IV. A spot test peel in these patients can rule in or rule out the possibility of postinflammatory hyperpigmentation or ultimate hypopigmentation.

A patient who is a heavy smoker, insulin-dependent diabetic, with a history of past radiation exposure to the face, or a patient with a collagen vascular disorder may not be a candidate for a resurfacing procedure. Spot test peel in these individuals can likewise confirm the ability of these individuals to reepithelialize normally. A patient who is hesitant to have a chemical peel because of a fear of an undesirable outcome can likewise be reassured by performing a spot test peel.

One should not be misled by the results of a spot test peel by the normal reepithelialization process and lack of postinflammatory hyperpigmentation or hypopigmentation because, whereas a test spot may heal perfectly, when a full-face chemical peel is performed, there can be pigmentary or textural changes simply because of the larger area that has been resurfaced. The spot test peel is, however, a good prognosticator of the ultimate outcome.

How do you handle peels in advanced Fitzpatrick skin types III, IV, V?

CORTEZ

Depending on their genealogy, some type III patients are suitable candidates for modified croton oil–phenol peeling. Olive-skinned, Mediterranean skin types are best treated with another modality. Black and Asian patients are not good candidates due to skin with a predilection for blotchy hyperpigmentation with areas of hypopigmentation. It should be noted that types I and II, who are typically highly freckled, may not be good candidates because of skin transition problems. I, personally, have treated many patients with type III skin with excellent results. Again, patient's family history and patient's personal history are extremely important in final evaluation.

FEDOK

In my practice, deeper peels such as the Baker-Gordon phenol based are only offered to patients with Fitzpatrick I and II skin types. These patients are also informed and counseled that the side effects of chemical peeling with this agent can be hyperpigmentation and hypopigmentation. In fact, they are told that they will most likely experience mild hypopigmentation of their skin.

I have not offered chemical peeling with the Baker-Gordon phenol based peels to patients with Fitzpatrick IV and V skin types. In selected patients with these skin types I have offered fractionated CO_2 and fractionated erbium resurfacing.

I have offered 35% TCA and 35% TCA plus Jessner solution peels[18,19] to selected patients with Fitzpatrick III and IV skin types. These patients are approached cautiously and counseled regarding the risk of hyperpigmentation. In my practice these patients are pretreated for 2 to 6 weeks with hydroquinone and retinoid creams, then restarted after they are reepithelialized. Using this rigid schedule I have not had any significant hyperpigmentation or hypopigmentation occur post procedure.

MANGAT

These higher Fitzpatrick skin types fortunately do not present with a same amount of actinic damage as do Fitzpatrick skin types I and II. It is rare to see medium or deep rhytids in any part of the face with the higher skin types. Skin type III may at times demonstrate fine periorbital or perioral rhytids. The majority of the time, these higher skin types display the presence of lentigines, dyschromia, and superficial to deep acne scars. Once again, the advent of the Hetter croton oil chemical peel formulas offers a distinct advantage for the higher skin types that was not present with the Baker-Gordon formula. One can more certainly perform a chemical peel using up to 0.4% croton oil concentration on a Fitzpatrick type III skin without fear of pigmentary changes. It must be mentioned that delayed epithelialization or scarring is no different in the higher skin types than in Fitzpatrick skin types I and II.

In order to avoid postinflammatory hyperpigmentation in these higher skin types, it is beneficial to pretreat these individuals with a hydroquinone formulation for approximately 4 to 6 weeks prior to the resurfacing procedure. I choose to use a preparation that consists of 8% hydroquinone, 1% hydrocortisone, and 0.05% retinoic acid in an emollient cream base. This preparation is applied on the areas to be treated twice a day for 4 to 6 weeks and restarted approximately 3 weeks following the chemical peel as long as the peeled areas are completely epithelialized. The use of this hydroquinone preparation in the postpeel period significantly diminishes the risk of postinflammatory hyperpigmentation.

It is interesting to note that melasma that has been resistant to improvement after the use of lighter chemical peels, kojic acid, hydroquinone, or intense pulsed light (IPL) can be treated a

0.1% or 0.2% Hetter peel or a straight USP 89% phenol solution with excellent resolution in any skin type.

The higher skin types III, IV, and V usually present for a resurfacing procedure because of the presence of acne scars rather than actinic damage. No matter what resurfacing modality is used on these individuals, there is a definite risk of temporary postinflammatory hyperpigmentation or permanent hypopigmentation. That risk has to be weighed against the severity of the scars and the individual's desire to have the scars improved regardless of pigmentary changes in the postresurfacing period. If such a patient is considered a candidate for dermabrasion or laser resurfacing as a modality to improve acne scars, then they are an equally good candidate for a croton oil–phenol chemical peel because the latter can be very effectively used to treat certain types of acne scars because of the potential for collagen enhancement and reorganization. The surgeon has to discuss the pigmentary changes that may result from a chemical peel for these patients and their willingness to resort to the use of makeup should there be significant hypopigmentation. Judicious use of a hydroquinone preparation, kojic acid, or IPL treatment can easily prevent or treat any postinflammatory hyperpigmentation that may occur in the higher skin types.

Postinflammatory hyperpigmentation will usually have its onset at 3 to 6 weeks after complete reepithelialization has occurred, which makes it essential that all of these peel patients are followed on a weekly basis after the peel for approximately 6 to 8 weeks. Early detection of postinflammatory hyperpigmentation will allow adequate treatment with a good outcome. As previously mentioned, postinflammatory hyperpigmentation is easily treated with judicious and aggressive means whereas hypopigmentation is irreversible and permanent. The latter makes it absolutely essential that the advanced Fitzpatrick skin types be very carefully counseled preoperatively to determine their willingness to use camouflage makeup should they develop hypopigmentation because there is no other solution for this problem. From a technique standpoint, it is absolutely imperative that every patient who undergoes any kind of chemical peel should have the border of the mandible marked in the sitting position prior to performing the peel and the peeling agent be used to feather into the neck past the border of the mandible in order to avoid a very sharp line of demarcation should hypopigmentation be an eventuality. It goes without saying that all peel patients regardless of skin type be treated with pre- and postpeel antiviral agents to avoid a herpetic outbreak in the peeled area, which can be devastating.

What is the main factor for rate of reepithelialization: (1) depth of peel, (2) depth of laser, (3) depth of dermabrasion?

CORTEZ

Assuming that we are trying to ablate medium and deep rhytids, deep resurfacing is defined as injury to the upper reticular dermis. This can be done with the phenol–croton oil peel, laser resurfacing, or dermabrasion. Although treatment with all of these modalities usually leads to reepithelialization in 7 to 14 days, depending on the residual adenexa, dermal thickening and collagen production does not begin until the inflammatory reaction subsides (**Fig. 7**).

Reepithelialization is the trademark of wound healing, but can be related to factors other than merely depth of the wounding modality. These partial-thickness wounds penetrate partially, but not deeply, into the dermis, and these injuries heal by reepithelialization from adenexa epithelium.

A major factor in wound reepithelialization is the epithelial migration rate, which is strongly affected by water content of the wound. Medium and deep wounding modalities reepithelialize most rapidly when they are maximally hydrated. Maibach and Rovee, in their elegant studies, showed unequivocally how much faster a wound heals when kept constantly moist. Thus, adequate and persistent hydration of the wound with petrolatum-based agents will markedly increase the rate of reepithelialization. Allowing wounds of this nature to desiccate will result in delayed healing and increased rate of scar formation.

Another issue that needs to be discussed is epidermal skin treatments prior to ablative therapies. We take patients off of all agents that might

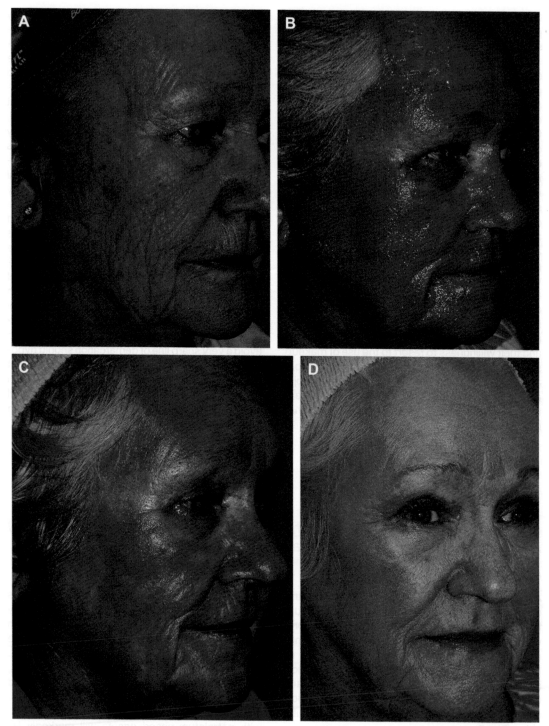

Fig. 7. Cortez. (*A*) Before peel. (*B*) Postoperative day 7. (*C*) Postoperative day 14. (*D*) One year postoperatively.

affect epidermal kinetics 1 month prior to surgery. We feel that use of retinoids, α- and β-hydroxy acids, and other exfoliating agents might possibly affect peel depth. Since we scrub the stratum corneum prior to peeling, we choose not to add another variable, which might affect our ablative technique. We realize that other authors feel that skin preparation with retinoids prior to resurfacing, in contrast, increases the rate of reepithelialization.

FEDOK

The rate of reepithelialization is multifactorial. One can expect patients undergoing procedures with less aggressive modalities to heal and reepithelialize in less time than those undergoing treatment with more aggressive modalities. For example, one usually expects the patient undergoing the medium-depth 35% TCA and Jessner solution peel to heal faster than the patient undergoing the Baker-Gordon formula phenol-based peel. The depth of injury is not only related to the agent itself, but is also related to the surgeon's technique in applying the peel solution.

In a parallel fashion, one can usually expect the patient undergoing fractionated erbium or fractionated CO_2 lasering to heal quicker than the patient undergoing full ablative CO_2 lasering. Those undergoing a superficial dermabrasion such as by the use of a diamond fraise will heal more rapidly than the patient undergoing a deeper dermabrasion by the use of a wire brush. The rapidity of reepithelialization or healing is conversely related to the depth of injury of the skin created by the applied technique.

The deeper the injury, the slower the healing. The more superficial the injury, the more rapid the healing. The beneficial effects are also related to the depth of injury. The deeper the injury, the more changes in the skin are produced. The more superficial the injury, the fewer changes in the skin are produced. Finally, the risk of complications also increases as the depth of injury increases.

Although the depth of injury may be the dominant factor in determining the rate of healing, it is not the only factor. Other factors that are within the realm of influence of the surgeon include whether or not the patient has undergone any pharmacologic skin conditioning before the procedure. In my practice we generally pretreat the patients with retinoids and hydroquinone. The effectiveness of these preconditioning maneuvers, however, is controversial. The postoperative care also affects the rate of reepithelialization. It has been demonstrated that the use of moist occlusive dressings promote wound healing. There are a variety of different ointments and occlusive dressings used, some commercial and some proprietary. In our practice we simply recommend the use of Vaseline, Aquaphor, Eucerin cream and, oddly enough, Preparation H. These dressings are interspersed with the application of mild acetic acid compresses. In our practice it has become clinically evident that the patients are more comfortable and the skin heals quicker if the patients use an adequate amount of ointment.

In carrying out a chemical peel, active degreasing of the patient's skin with acetone and a gauze pad is commonly done to remove skin oils and to promote agent penetration. Depending on the vigorousness of the degreasing, one can actually be performing a mild dermabrasion or exfoliation of the skin with the gauze pad, rather than a simple degreasing. This "degreasing" action does become a variable part of the peeling procedure, and influences the depth of penetration and effect of the peeling agent. Finally, the state of the skin itself and the overall health of the patient each influence the rate of healing.

In summary, although the depth of injury is probably the most significant factor affecting healing time, there are several other important factors.

MANGAT

There are several factors that determine the rate of epithelialization following a chemical peel, laser resurfacing, or dermabrasion, and they are as follows:

1. The depth of the resurfacing that is performed regardless of the entity that is used determines how quickly the treated area will reepithelialize. Resurfacing modalities will penetrate either

through the epidermis, through the papillary dermis, or down to the reticular dermis. When penetrating just through the epidermis, reepithelialization will usually occur within 5 days; when going down to the papillary dermis, it is 7 days; and when going to the reticular dermis it can take 7 to 14 days for reepithelialization to occur.

2. How the resurfaced area is treated determines to a significant extent the rate of reepithelialization. Using a dry occlusive dressing such as Xeroform as with dermabrasion, there can be a slightly prolonged period for reepithelialization as opposed to using a wet dressing such as petrolatum type of ointment, antibiotic ointment, or an emollient cream such as Eucerin.

When using a wet dressing on the resurfaced area, reepithelialization is usually faster because it prevents the formation of a crust and the moist surface heals faster.

3. It is my experience that when using laser resurfacing, reepithelialization can be longer than with a chemical peel or dermabrasion, and this may possibly be related to adjacent thermal damage from the laser that is not seen with chemical peel or dermabrasion.

4. General health factors such as a history of smoking, diabetes, and microvascular disease, cardiovascular disease, or other systemic illness may have an influence on the rate of reepithelialization.

Analysis: how has your approach to or technique in chemical peels evolved over the past several years?

Dr Cortez provides a narrated video of croton peel application.

CORTEZ

For years, the gold standard in ablative resurfacing for medium and deep rhytids has been the Baker-Gordon peel. However, the theories of its action appear to have been based on misinformation. The concept that phenol was the only active ingredient and that croton oil was only a slight irritant that could be omitted has been dispelled since the early 1990s. With the studies of both Hetter and Stone, we modified the classic Baker-Gordon peel into a resurfacing spectrum by varying the amount of croton oil in each formula.

Selecting the correct formula for the appropriate skin type, skin damage, and facial zone provides the ability to maximize the results and minimize the complications. The strict adherence to detailed preoperative preparation, formula preparation and selection, and postoperative care and follow-up has shown consistently superior results.

In conclusion, some of our most happy and grateful patients in the short and long term are those who have been resurfaced with our croton oil–phenol preparation (**Fig. 8**).

FEDOK

In our practice we offer a simple spectrum of resurfacing techniques to patients. The spectrum offered is:

- Medium-depth 35% TCA and Jessner solution chemical peel
- Baker-Gordon phenol-based chemical peel
- Fractionated erbium laser
- Fractionated CO_2 laser
- Full ablative CO_2 laser

This array of procedures offers patients with a variety skin types and skin aging a reasonable selection of options. This group of

techniques represents a spectrum of depth of injury, effectiveness, potential side effects and complications, and downtime. The patient depicted in **Fig. 9**A and B has undergone a Baker-Gordon Peel, the patient in Fig. 9C and D has undergone a 35% trichloracetic acid and Jessner's solution peel.

The majority of our patients are placed on a preconditioning or pretreatment regimen prior to their resurfacing procedure. Depending on scheduling, the duration of this preconditioning is 2 to 4 weeks. The regimen that we utilize with most patients includes the use of retinoids and hydroquinone. These are stopped 2 days before

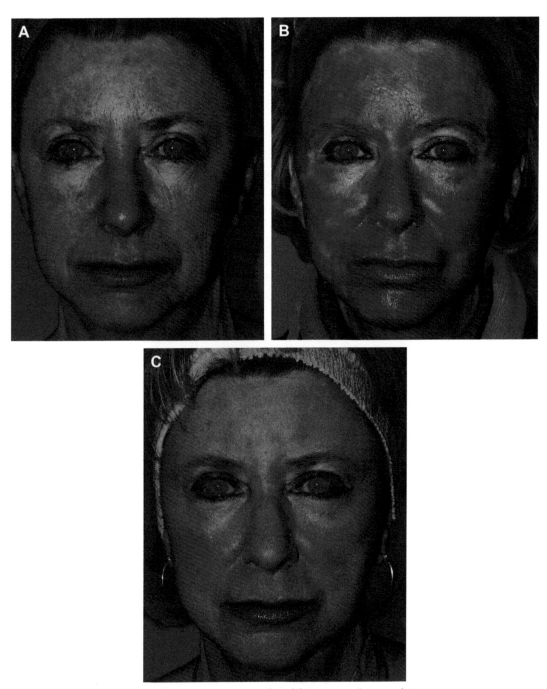

Fig. 8. Cortez. (A) Before peel. (B) Postoperative month 1. (C) Postoperative month 7.

the procedures. This is done whether the patient is undergoing a laser or a chemical peel procedure.

All patients, regardless of resurfacing modality, are given a variety of oral medications including antibacterial antibiotics and, even more importantly, antivirals in the perioperative period. The antivirals are started 2 days before the procedure and continued for 14 days after the procedure.

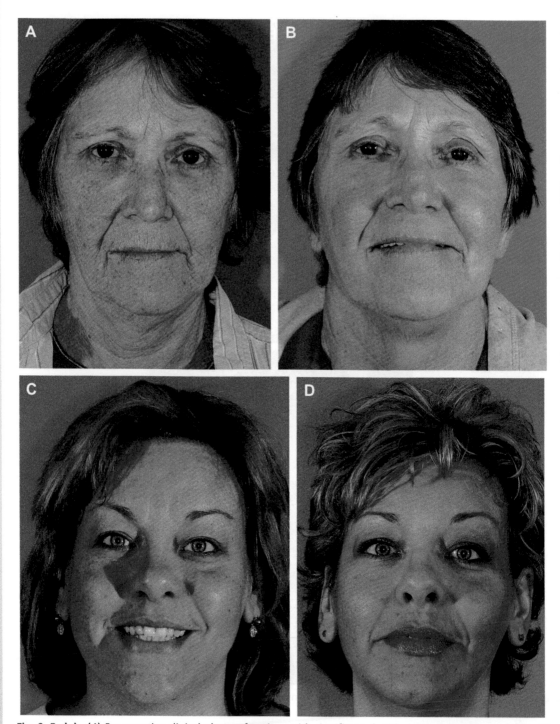

Fig. 9. Fedok. (*A*) Preoperative clinical photo of patient with significant rhytids, lentigines, and skin laxity. (*B*) Same patient as in *A* 6 months after full-face Baker-Gordon peel. Note improvement in skin texture, pigmentation, and laxity. (*C*) Preoperative clinical photo of patient with rhytids and mild lentigines. (*D*) Same patient as in *C* after full-face 35% trichloroacetic acid (TCA)/Jessner solution peel. Note improvement in skin texture, lentigines, and fine rhytids.

In order to further customize their treatment, patients are frequently managed with a "combination" peel in which they undergo a deeper peel in the areas with more significant rhytids and a superficial peel in less affected areas. This is usually reserved for patients with Fitzpatrick I and II skin types. The method of using a combination such as this allows treatment of the patient's entire facial area while avoiding some of the morbidity and downtime of a full-face deep chemical peel (**Fig. 10**). The postoperative care regimen was briefly touched on earlier, and is shown in **Table 1**. Patients are closely monitored for infection, hyperpigmentation, hypopigmentation, and prolonged erythema. After reepithelialization the patients may begin their retinoid creams again and, depending on their progress, they may be additionally treated with hydroquinone and steroid creams.

MANGAT

Over the past 5 years or slightly longer, my technique for chemical peels has evolved significantly, having stopped performing the standard Baker-Gordon chemical peel and changing to the varied

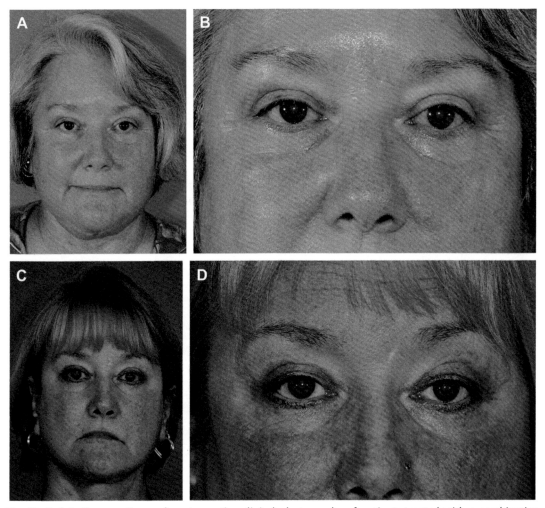

Fig. 10. Fedok. Preoperative and postoperative clinical photographs of patients treated with a combination Baker-Gordon and 35% TCA/Jessner peel. (*A–D*) Preoperative (*A, B*) and postoperative (*C, D*) views of a patient whose periorbital area was treated with the Baker-Gordon peel and the remainder of the face treated with 35% TCA/Jessner peel.

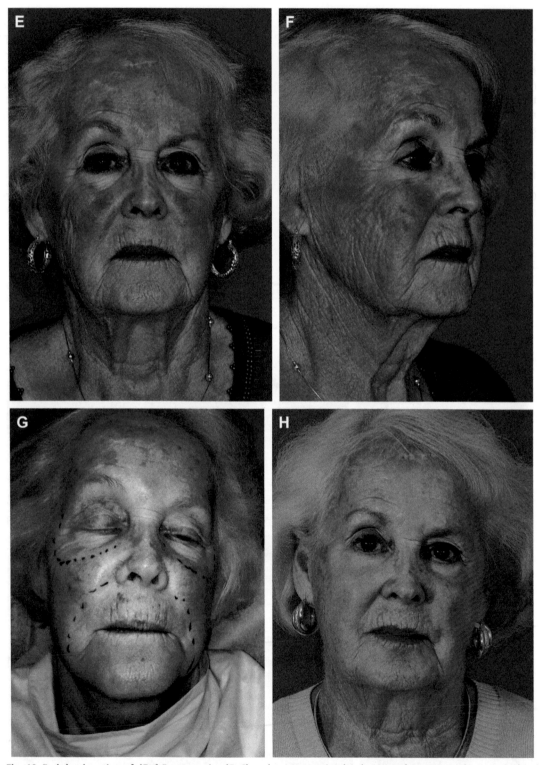

Fig. 10. Fedok. (*continued*) (*E–J*) Preoperative (*E–G*) and postoperative (*H–J*) views of a patient whose periorbital area and perioral areas were treated with the Baker-Gordon peel and the remainder of the face treated with 35% TCA/Jessner peel.

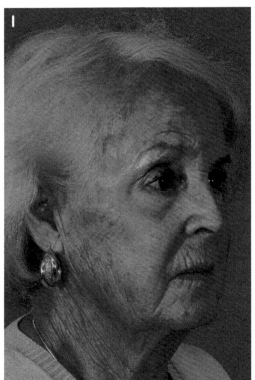

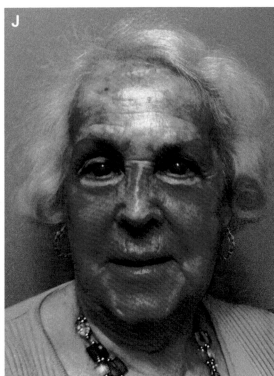

Fig. 10. Fedok. (*continued*)

croton oil concentration Hetter chemical peel, thus having better control of the depth of the peel determined by the nature of the skin and the extent of actinic damage on different parts of the face. Adopting this change has allowed me to be able to offer chemical peels to a wider spectrum of patients with predictable and consistent results, having significantly minimized some of the undesirable sequelae of the more aggressive older Baker-Gordon chemical peel. The incidence of hypopigmentation has been virtually eliminated and the healing time, particularly the extent of erythema after the peel, has also been diminished significantly.

Having performed CO_2 laser resurfacing for approximately 5 years and then returning to the chemical peeling technique of skin resurfacing, the most important thing that I have learned in performing chemical peels is that one is still able to get very satisfactory results without subjecting my patients to a more aggressive chemical peeling process that not only prolongs the healing time, but also increases the risk of unsatisfactory sequelae. My goals for achieving change in a patient with actinic damage have changed to become more realistic and more in line with the patient's expectations of bringing about significant improvement but not complete elimination of all rhytids in the face. My patients who have extensive actinic damage with deep rhytids and severe dyschromia are quite accepting of the fact that all rhytids may not be completely eliminated and that they would obtain a pleasing result even though some rhytids may exist to a fine degree.

In summary, the Hetter chemical peel technique has shifted my thinking from an idealistic approach to a more realistic goal, without compromising the patient's expectations and final outcome.

Table 1
Fedok. Postpeel instructions

Section: Postoperative Care of Chemical Peels, Lasers, and Dermabrasions	
	Please follow these instructions carefully. You should also review the materials relative to your surgery. Your final result will depend upon how well you care for the treated areas
	Notify our office if any rash or fever blister-like areas should appear
Week 1 (beginning the day after surgery)	Spray plain lukewarm water 6 times daily on affected areas while using fingertips to pat skin (showering is preferable). This should be done 5–10 min each time depending on size of areas involved. Pat skin dry with Kleenex brand unscented tissues. Apply Vaseline. Eucerine Cream (or other cream _____ as directed by your physician) to skin with fingers. (Apply only to treated areas.) Use a gentle massaging motion when applying cream. Apply enough cream to keep your new skin and any crusting soft. Use Kleenex brand unscented tissues to blot or soak up excess cream from skin before each cleansing with water
	DO NOT use a washcloth or towel on the treated areas. DO NOT rub your new skin with fingers between treatments. DO NOT use heavy applications of cream. DO NOT rub or wipe skin with Kleenex. DO NOT use cotton balls or Q-tips on the treated areas
Week 2	Continue cleansing as above if crusts are still present. Use the creams as directed by the doctor if cleansing is continued. Keep areas "moisturized" with the recommended cream at all times
Week 3	You may use water-based hypoallergenic makeup if your skin is smooth and free of crusts. Remove makeup in shower with water only. Use the recommended cream under base makeup as a moisturizer
Week 4	Use Neutrogena soap (Original Formula) to cleanse skin. Rinse thoroughly to remove soap film
	DO NOT use any other soaps, moisturizers, cleansing creams, Retin-A, etc on face until you have been instructed to do so
Week 5	You may use oil-based makeup, if desired. Use at least a #30 sunscreen to protect face against sun exposure. "Test" a small area before using sunscreen on the entire area being treated. Resume reasonable physical activities
DO NOT use sunscreen if irritation occurs. DO NOT use Retin-A anywhere on face or body if irritation occurs.	
ASK YOUR DOCTOR if you have questions about when to resume these products and makeup.	
Remember, your new skin is as sensitive and delicate as a newborn baby's…so…use good judgment. As healing progresses, your new skin will become more resilient, but, this may take 3–6 mo. Most people agree that the final results are worth the inconvenience.	

SUPPLEMENTARY DATA

Supplementary data related to this article can be found online at http://dx.doi.org/10.1016/j.fsc.2013.09.004.

REFERENCES: FEDOK

1. Ridenour BD. Insights in Otolaryngology 1993;8(6): 1–11.
2. Bailey AJ, Robins SP, Balin G. Biological significance of the intermolecular crosslinks of collagen. Nature 1974;251:105–9.
3. Daly CH, Odland GF. Age-related changes in the mechanical properties of human skin. J Invest Dermatol 1979;73:84–7.
4. Kligman AM. Perspectives and problems in cutaneous gerontology. J Invest Dermatol 1979;73:39–46.

5. Miyahara T, Murai A, Tanaka T, et al. Age-related differences in human skin collagen solubility in solvent, susceptibility to pepsin digestion, and the spectrum of the solubilized polymeric collagen molecules. J Gerontol 1982;37:651–5.

6. Leveque JL, Corcuff P, de Riga1 J, et al. In vivo studies of the evaluation of physical properties of the human skin with age. Int J Dermatol 1984;23:322–9.

7. Glogau RG. Aesthetic and anatomic analysis of the aging skin. Semin Cutan Med Surg 1996;15(3):134–8.

8. Langsdon PR, Milburn M, Yarber R. Comparison of the laser and phenol chemical peel in facial skin resurfacing. Arch Otolaryngol Head Neck Surg 2000;126(10):1195–9.

9. McCollough EG, Hillman RA Jr. Chemical face peel. Otolaryngol Clin North Am 1980;13(2):353–65.

10. McCollough EG, Langsdon PR. The maskless chemical face peel. Dermatol Clin 1987;5(2):381–92.

11. Truppman F, Ellenbery J. The major electrocardiographic changes during chemical face peeling. Plast Reconstr Surg 1979;63:44.

12. Wexler MR, Halon DA, Teitelbaum A, et al. The prevention of cardiac arrhythmias produced in an animal model by topical application of a phenol preparation in common use for face peeling. Plast Reconstr Surg 1984;73:595–8.

13. Litton C, Trinidad G. Complications of chemical face peeling as evaluated by a questionnaire. Plast Reconstr Surg 1981;67:738–44.

14. Brody HJ. Complications of chemical peels. In: Brody HJ, editor. Chemical peeling and resurfacing. 2nd edition. St Louis (MO): Mosby; 1997. p. 187–9.

15. Gross BG. Cardiac arrhythmias during phenol face peeling. Plast Reconstr Surg 1984;73:590–4.

16. Price NM. EKG changes in relationship to the chemical peel. J Dermatol Surg Oncol 1990;16:37–42.

17. Botta SA, Straith RE, Goodwin HH. Cardiac arrhythmias in phenol face peeling: a suggested protocol for prevention. Aesthetic Plast Surg 1988;12:115–7.

18. Monheit GD. Advances in chemical peeling. Facial Plast Surg Clin North Am 1994;2:5–9.

19. Monheit GD. The Jessner's-TCA peel. Facial Plast Surg Clin North Am 1994;2:21–2.

CORTEZ RECOMMENDED READINGS

Baker T, Stuzin J, Baker T. Facial skin resurfacing. St. Louis (MO): QMP; 1998.

Brody JH, editor. Chemical peeling. St. Louis (MO): Mosby; 1997.

Hetter GP. An examination of phenol-croton oil peel: part IV. Face peel results with different concentrations of phenol and croton oil. Plast Reconstr Surg 2000;105(3):1061–83.

Rubin M, editor. Chemical peels. Philadelphia: Elsevier Saunders; 2006.

Stone PA, Lefer L. Modified phenol chemical face peels: recognizing the role of application technique. Facial Plast Surg Clin North Am 2001;9(3):351–76.

MANGAT SUGGESTED READINGS

Brody HJ. Complications of chemical peeling. J Dermatol Surg Oncol 1989;15:1010–9.

Brody HJ. Variations and comparisons in medium depth chemical peeling. J Dermatol Surg Oncol 1989;15:953–63.

Garlich PH, Mangat DS. Advances in chemical peels: modified phenol-croton oil medium depth peels. Advanced Therapy in Facial Plastic and Reconstructive Surgery. Chapter 49.

Hetter GP. An examination of the croton oil peel: part I. Dissecting the formula. Plast Reconstr Surg 2000;105:227–39.

Hetter GP. An examination of the croton oil peel: part II. The lay peelers and their croton oil formulas. Plast Reconstr Surg 2000;105:240–8.

Hetter GP. An examination of the phenol-croton oil peel: part III. The plastic surgeons role. Plast Reconstr Surg 2000;105(2):752–63.

Hetter GP. An examination of the phenol-croton oil peel: part IV. Face peel results with different concentrations of the phenol and croton oil. Plast Reconstr Surg 2000;105(3):1061–83.

Monheig GD. Advances in chemical peeling. Facial Plast Surg Clin North Am 1994;2:5–9.

Stegman SJ. A comparative histologic study of the effects of three peeling agents and dermabrasion on normal and sun damaged skin. Aesthetic Plast Surg 1982;6:123–35.

Stone PA, Lefer LG. Modified phenol chemical based peels: recognizing the role of application technique. Facial Plast Surg Clin North Am 2001;9(3):351–76.

Rhinoplasty: Panel Discussion

Peter A. Adamson, MD[a,b],*, Minas Constantinides, MD[c],*,
Alyn J. Kim, MD[a,b],*, Steven Pearlman, MD[d,e],*

KEYWORDS

- Rhinoplasty • Alloplastic implant • Spreader graft • Tip-plasty

---

Rhinoplasty Panel Discussion

Minas Constantinides, Peter Adamson, Alyn Kim, and Steven Pearlman address questions for discussion and debate:

1. Should one use an open or closed rhinoplasty approach?
2. How appropriate is the endonasal approach in modern-day rhinoplasty?
3. Should the tip lobule be divided or preserved?
4. Are alloplastic implants inferior to autologous implants?
5. Does release and reduction of the upper lateral cartilages from the nasal dorsal septum always require spreader graft placement to prevent mid one-third nasal pinching in reduction rhinoplasty?
6. *Analysis*: over the past 5 years, how has your technique or approach evolved or what is the most important thing you've learned in doing rhinoplasty?

CONSTANTINIDES: INTRODUCTION

Theory without practice is like a one-winged bird that is incapable of flight.
—*Sushruta medical writings, India, 600 BC*

Science is the father of knowledge, but opinion breeds ignorance.
—*Hippocrates, Kos, Greece, 400 BC*

I am an open rhinoplasty surgeon. Since entering practice in 1994, I have performed over 2000 primary and revision open rhinoplasties. As Director of Facial Plastic and Reconstructive Surgery in the Department of Otolaryngology at New York University School of Medicine, I teach and operate at NYU Langone Medical Center, Bellevue Hospital Center, and the Manhattan Veterans Administration Hospital. From my first day in practice I have been a rhinoplasty teacher. I have taught 19 years' worth of residents open rhinoplasty, and many have gone on to perform rhinoplasty in their practices. In 2000 I started a fellowship in Facial Plastic Surgery. I included Drs Norman Pastorek and Philip Miller in order to give my fellows a wide array of exposure to various approaches in rhinoplasty (in addition to all other aspects of facial plastic surgery). I recognize the importance of

---

Disclaimer: Dr Peter A. Adamson is on the Physician Advisory Board for Allergan Canada.
[a] Adamson Cosmetic Facial Surgery Inc., M110 - 150 Bloor Street West, Toronto, Ontario M5S 2X9, Canada;
[b] Department of Otolaryngology - Head and Neck Surgery, University Health Network, University of Toronto, Toronto, Ontario, Canada; [c] Department of Otolaryngology, New York University School of Medicine & New York Head & Neck Institute, New York, NY, USA; [d] Columbia University, New York, NY, USA; [e] Center for Aesthetic Facial Surgery, New York Head and Neck Institute, Manhattan Eye Ear and Throat Hospital, Lenox Hill Hospital, Northshore-L I J Hospital System, New York, NY, USA
* Corresponding authors. Adamson Cosmetic Facial Surgery, Inc., M110 – 150 Bloor Street West Toronto, Ontario, Canada M5S 2×9 (Adamson); 74 East 79th Street, Suite 1-B, New York, NY 10075 (Constantinides); Facial Plastic and Reconstructive Surgery, 521 Park Avenue, New York, NY 10065 (Pearlman).
E-mail addresses: paa@dradamson.com (Adamson); drconstantinides@gmail.com (Constantinides); drpearlman@mdface.com (Pearlman)

facialplastic.theclinics.com

seeing a variety of surgeons handle a variety of problems in unique ways. I could think of no one better to teach closed rhinoplasty that Dr Pastorek, probably the best closed surgeon in the world today.

The controversies discussed in this *Clinics* issue are well chosen to reflect how my own philosophy has changed over my years in practice. In my answers, I hope to paint a picture of how I decide to do what I do in rhinoplasty today, why I have changed what I do over the years and how even now I am looking for better ways to improve what I do. Dr Eugene Tardy has said, "the rhinoplasty student never graduates." This complex and beautiful operation is at once rewarding and humbling. I am blessed that my practice is a rhinoplasty practice on such a large and demanding stage.

Should one use an open or closed rhinoplasty approach?

ADAMSON AND KIM

Open septorhinoplasty (OSR) was introduced 40 years ago in North America and has since gained wide acceptance as a good approach, if not the preferred approach, for rhinoplasty. In a survey by Dayan and Kanodia of fellowship graduates of the American Academy of Facial Plastic and Reconstructive Surgery between 1997 and 2007, they found that the vast majority, 87.9%, performed open rhinoplasty as their primary approach.[1] The open approach to rhinoplasty has been controversial since its inception, but this statistic indicates increasingly wide acceptance of this approach.[2] In the past, open rhinoplasty was supported for difficult or revision cases only. Proponents of closed rhinoplasty initially criticized the open technique, citing potential problems such as unnecessary scarring, reduction of tip support, extended operative time, and excessive postoperative tip swelling. The issue of columellar scarring was addressed by Vuyk and Olde Kalter[3] in a meta-analysis of 7 articles encompassing 986 patients who underwent open septorhinoplasty. Only 3 had columellar flap necrosis that led to scarring. Another argument against OSR was that the open scar was longer when, in fact, it, and the marginal incision, are shorter than the scars of a cartilage delivery technique and do not affect the internal valve, an area of potential functional compromise in closed approaches.[4] Other potential arguments against the open approach are purportedly longer lasting supratip swelling and longer operative times. Toriumi and colleagues[5] used cadaver studies to demonstrate that the main vasculature of the nose runs aloft the musculoaponeurotic layer, or in it and parallel to the alar margin, as opposed to vertically in the columella. Thus, it is dissection above the musculoaponeurotic layer that disrupts and perhaps prolongs postoperative tip edema, not the transcolumellar incision of OSR. Indeed, operative times may be longer with OSR because more time may be taken to deal with the asymmetries that are uncovered.

The open approach clearly offers better exposure to a small surgical field, thereby affording the opportunity to better diagnose the deformity through inspection, to better execute certain maneuvers, and to teach and to learn the operation with greater ease.[6–8] Indications have expanded with widespread increasing levels of comfort and familiarity with the technique. In my experience, open rhinoplasty is the technique of choice for all cases unless a comparable improvement for a definable deformity can be obtained with the closed approach. The open approach offers clear diagnostic and therapeutic advantages for many challenging functional and cosmetic nasal deformities, primarily resulting from the broad undistorted exposure it affords and the improved opportunity for bimanual correction. This is especially true with respect to the premaxillary spine, caudal septum, dorsal and superior septum, lobule, and superior dorsum. The open approach offers an unparalleled appreciation of the underlying anatomy resulting in the external deformity. Sutures can be placed, grafts trimmed exactly, and asymmetries corrected without distortion of surrounding tissues. Scar tissue and redundant subcutaneous tissue are more easily excised. The valve region can be well protected, and the absence of incisions in the intercartilaginous region diminishes subsequent obstructive phenomena by precluding scar formation and disruption of one of the tip support mechanisms. It may also be that revision rates for primary OSR are less than those for closed rhinoplasty.[9,10]

OSR provides an opportunity for greater surgical exposure for the operating surgeon and the assistants, and thereby provides an excellent teaching tool. As this approach is used in didactic teaching sessions, more surgeons in training are exposed to the approach and may be more apt to continue with this approach in their later practices. In general, surgeons with the greatest experience (more than 100 rhinoplasties per year) tend to use the closed approach more often, but, nonetheless, even they still perform a notable amount of OSR. There is still some trend to increasing use of the OSR approach: the only group using it slightly less are those in practice 16 to 25 years—older surgeons who were less exposed to the OSR approach in their training and continue to practice in the manner in which they were trained. Younger surgeons perform open rhinoplasty more frequently compared with older surgeons for all indications.[11] The movement toward open rhinoplasty seems to be plateauing with possibly a slight upward trend in its use. Except for "simple" cases, OSR may be indicated for rhinoplasty by a large proportion of surgeons, especially for rhinoplasties that are "difficult" or revisions or those requiring grafting. When all is said and done, each surgeon will assess the patient's deformity and their own ability to correct it, and will utilize the approach that works best for them. There will always be room for differing opinions and different approaches.

CONSTANTINIDES

Note: Constantinides here discusses open versus closed approach jointly with the next discussion of endonasal approach.

When discussing open and closed approaches, the terms themselves engender controversy. "Open" is also called "external" while "closed" is called "endonasal." Should one set of terms be abandoned for another? There are good arguments on both sides. In favor of keeping "open" and "closed" are the arguments that:

- "Closed" correctly characterizes the approach as obscured, with inferior visualization and poor ability to exactly manipulate cartilages in their native position.
- "External" correctly characterizes the trivial columellar incision as being of consequence. It is not.
- It is simpler for a patient to say and to remember "open" and "closed."

In favor of using "external" and "endonasal":

- "Closed" was called "closed" only when the "open" approach was introduced.
- "Closed" implies without incisions, as in "closed reduction of a nasal fracture."
- "Endonasal" correctly refers to an approach with incisions only inside the nose.

Historical perspective is important. The open approach was used in Germany by Johann Friedrich Diffenbach who described a dorsal midline vertical incision in his "Die Operative Chirurgie" in 1845. Jacques Joseph's first case in 1898 used the same approach, but he later switched to an endonasal approach to avoid the scar. He thought he was first to perform an endonasal rhinoplasty, but had been beaten by two New York surgeons. John Orlando Roe reported the first endonasal rhinoplasty in 1887[1] and Robert F. Weir reported his first in 1892 (although he claimed he had performed it in 1885 in order to beat Roe).[2]

What does a Google search reveal on "Open versus Closed Rhinoplasty"?[3] The #1 position is held by Dr Steven M. Denenberg, who lists a number of conditions that must exist for him to use the closed approach. He summarizes by saying: "I use the closed technique only about 5% of the time."[4] Other positions by other surgeons (some well-known, others not) essentially summarize the arguments that I have listed in often colorful (and sometimes misleading) language that captures each surgeon's individual sentiments on the subject. On the Web, the "open versus closed" argument is used as a publicity tool to scare patients away from one approach or the other, depending upon each surgeon's bias. Is there any wonder there is so much disinformation and confusion on this topic in the public's eye?

Since this issue of *Clinics* is to capture each expert's description of his particular approach, I will limit myself to a description of my open approach. I only use the closed approach in very minor revisions and never in primary rhinoplasty. Unlike Dr Denenberg, I have never found a primary rhinoplasty in which I do not want to fully visualize the entire nose. Even for relatively simple changes, the open approach allows me the possibility of hitting a home run. With the closed approach, I am worried that I will not have accounted for some unnoticed issue (cephalic excision releasing the lateral crus to become convex postop; minor dorsal reduction causing asymmetric upper lateral cartilage (ULC) weakness and postop irregularity) that could lead to a postoperative problem.

The incisions and the columellar scar
I use the same incision Goodman used when he introduced open rhinoplasty in Canada in 1979, the inverted "V" incision. The alternate incision,

the stair-step incision, I long thought was equivalent until I started having to revise it. There are several real problems with the stair-step. One is that the lateral limbs of the incision should be at the narrowest part of the columella. This is so that the incision is placed where the medial crura are closest to the skin. The underlying cartilage provides support against contraction, insuring the best possible resultant scar. Indeed, in columellas with thicker skin, I make sure that I reinforce the underlying cartilaginous support to insure a strong platform that resists contraction. The stair-step incision's lateral limbs are not ideally placed.

With the stair-step incision one limb is higher on one side of the columella than the other. If scar revision is required, excising the incision can leave one side of the resultant scar too close to the top of the columella, creating the potential for notching and nostril asymmetry. The inverted "V" incision forces the resultant limbs lower on the columella, so any subsequent scar revision is simpler and the chance for asymmetry is less (**Fig. 1**).

If performing scar revision, the resulting closing tension may be improved by extending the marginal incisions inferiorly toward the sill. The lower portion of the columella then may be dissected as an advancement flap, providing ample release and decreasing the closing tension. A single buried 5-0 Monocryl suture in the midline further reduces the chance of scar widening during the contraction phase of healing. Simple 6-0 nylon interrupted sutures placed to evert the skin edges create a nearly invisible scar.

Another variable when planning the open incision is the lateral extent of the marginal incision. In primary rhinoplasties, my marginal incisions now end where the caudal edges of the lateral crura diverge cephalically away from the rim. Extending the marginal incision more laterally does little to enhance exposure; the lateral crura may still be dissected in their entirety without a longer marginal incision. Limiting the length of the marginal incision has theoretic and practical benefits. Theoretically, there is less disruption of the lateral lymphatics and vascular drainage from the tip.[5] This may lead to less edema postoperatively and less chance of prolonged thickening of the soft tissue envelope. Practically, the shorter marginal incision allows more stability when placing rim grafts and batten grafts into pockets in this area.

Point of view The main practical difference between an open and a closed exposure is the point of view of the surgeon. From a closed exposure, the surgeon's point of view is from lateral to medial. When dissecting and then viewing the dissected structures, the surgeon looks from lateral to medial, whether looking through a marginal or an intercartilaginous incision. From this point of view, it is impossible to directly judge bilateral symmetry simultaneously. Instead, the closed surgeon must judge symmetry by viewing and palpating the nose externally through an already dissected soft tissue envelope. This may be why a skilled closed surgeon has such difficulty with the open approach. He is used to judging symmetry while looking from the outside. His eye is not used to judging symmetry by directly observing the dissected structures, especially when the transcolumellar incision has freed the skin envelope in a way he is not used to seeing.

The open approach affords a completely different point of view. Instead of dissecting and viewing from lateral to medial, the surgeon begins by dissecting symmetrically and bilaterally. The entire operation develops from a midline perspective. This makes the open approach exceptionally suited for creating symmetry from the midline. The direct exposure of nasal structures as they diverge from the midline allows the surgeon an

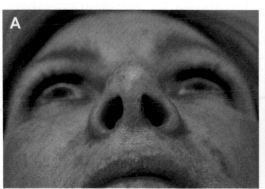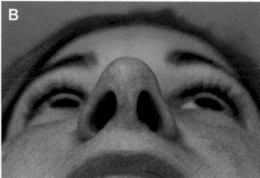

Fig. 1. Constantinides. (*A, B*) Typical inverted "V" columellar scars are barely invisible.

unparalleled view for creating a symmetric result. This is why an open surgeon has such difficulty with the closed approach. He is used to seeing the nasal structures from the top down, symmetrically and bilaterally. He is not used to judging symmetry by observing it from lateral to medial, and is not used to trusting what he sees when looking through a dissected soft tissue envelope. Most of the "rules" that surgeons have created about when to use the open or the closed approach have to do with this difference in surgical point of view.

PEARLMAN

I'm honored to have been asked to participate in this exciting format for this issue of *Facial Plastic Surgery Clinics*. I feel that it's important to preface my remarks by clarifying the topic. To begin, the correct terms are more appropriately labeled: "external" and "endonasal" approaches to rhinoplasty. Additionally the use of the conjunction "versus" implies a competition, or adversarial dispute among surgeons who choose, and surgeons who choose not to use a tiny incision across the columella. I will address this alleged controversy more specifically in the next section. Most important in nasal surgery is not which approach is used, but the understanding of nasal anatomy, the repertoire of surgical maneuvers, and the consequence of each of those surgical maneuvers. Actually seeing the nasal structures by using an external approach and peeling back the skin does not automatically impart an understanding of nasal anatomy and surgical technique; it only provides a better view.

In what many consider a landmark textbook, *Open Structure Rhinoplasty*, Johnson and Toriumi[1] built on the approach first described by Rethi,[2] revived by Padovan,[3] and brought to North America by Goodman.[4] The addition of the principle of "structure" is the key and the true genius of that simple phrase and book title. Structure must be maintained or restored in both external and endonasal rhinoplasty.

Emphasizing the importance of structure and its necessity for successful rhinoplasty follows the architectural dictum: "form follows function." Although this phrase was first coined by the mid-nineteenth century sculptor Horatio Greenough,[5] it has more commonly been applied to the modernist architecture movement of Louis Sullivan and his disciple Frank Lloyd Wright. Their German counterpart, the Bauhaus, espoused similar principles. When analyzing the appearance of a nose and proposing surgery, especially for revision rhinoplasty, I often bring up the concept of "form follows function." What doesn't look good in an overdone nose doesn't work well either. The reverse is true as well, what doesn't work well also doesn't look natural.

The surgical techniques we employ to make noses look better should also improve nasal function. Occasionally patients actually state that they don't care about their airway in deference to an improved appearance, which is heard more often during a revision rhinoplasty consultation. It should be pointed out that, unless they are seeking a tiny pinched nose, as was fashionable in the 1960s, both improved form and function can, and should, be addressed. What we are creating or restoring is a more attractive conduit that functions as a Starling resistor being acted on by Bernoulli forces. The nasal walls need the size and strength to resist the negative pressure due to air flow in the upper airway.

Maintaining or restoring nasal structure through the use of spreader grafts to support the middle vault was first proposed by Sheen[6] over a decade before Johnson, yet Sheen practiced exclusively endonasal surgery. Personally, I am now using spreader grafts in well over 90% of both primary and revision rhinoplasties through either the external or endonasal approach (see question below: *Are alloplastic implants inferior to autologous implants*?).

Structure is important for the external nasal vault as well. Over the past few decades we have been taught to leave increasingly more lateral crural height. Yet we still want more refined nasal tips. Tip narrowing or sculpting sutures can be used for additional refinement. Now that the importance of middle vault structure and support has been well established, authors have become increasingly aware of the complex contributions of the lateral crura to external valve form and function.[7–9]

Despite many advances in rhinoplasty over the past few decades the rate of revision rhinoplasty still hasn't changed.[10,11] Recently, I have found that the majority of revision rhinoplasties I perform are on external rhinoplasties, unless the

I am an open rhinoplasty surgeon. I have gotten accustomed to creating symmetric, stable results using a midline point of view. I admire my closed rhinoplasty colleagues who create exceptional results from another point of view, but I do not covet their approach. I know the open approach in my hands gives my patients the best chance for an exceptional result with the least chance of any asymmetry or irregularity. The columellar scar is inconsequential; no blog entry will convince me otherwise.

rhinoplasty was performed over 15 years ago. This is not a condemnation of that approach, but more likely due to the overwhelming majority of current practitioners using that approach. There are a number of questions that remain on the topic of revision rates. Is it that there are more surgeons attempting rhinoplasty? Are the patients becoming more sophisticated and exacting, or are the ideas of what constitutes an acceptable result in the eyes of both surgeons and patients more stringent than 2 decades ago? Does the open approach make rhinoplasty seem easier and more likely for the uninitiated surgeon to attempt? I would delve further, but this subject is more appropriate for another discussion.

I have strayed from the assigned question of open versus closed rhinoplasty. That is because it's less a controversy and more a choice. I know a number of very skilled surgeons who get superb results from both approaches.

How appropriate is the endonasal approach in modern-day rhinoplasty?

ADAMSON AND KIM

OSR has been found useful for most indications except for the "simple" tip or dorsum. The closed, or endonasal approaches continue to have their proponents, for very good reasons, and appear to be especially useful for the "simple" tip and dorsum. The most experienced surgeons may favor the closed approaches, but even they have initiated notable use of OSR. Perhaps the consensus opinion is best summed up by recognizing the challenging operation that rhinoplasty is and the unique training and experience that each rhinoplasty surgeon has. I recommend that each surgeon initially consider the open approach for a given case, unless the surgeon believes he or she can make the diagnosis and correct the deformities with a closed approach, in which case it can be used. I also recommend that rather than learning and less frequently applying a large number of approaches in one's armamentarium, a surgeon use as small a number of approaches as necessary and use them more frequently to achieve good results within one's experience. In this way, a surgeon increases his or her experience and becomes maximally adept at each.

CONSTANTINIDES

Readers are directed to Constantinides' responses to the previous question

PEARLMAN

The endonasal approach to rhinoplasty is absolutely appropriate in modern-day rhinoplasty if the surgeon is well trained in the procedure. Results from skilled surgeons are just as good as their counterparts who utilize the external approach exclusively.

Just stating this question actually counters the 2-decade-old contention about open versus closed rhinoplasty. I have heard it said that closed rhinoplasty is practiced with a closed mind and open rhinoplasty an open mind to a more modern technique. I feel the opposite may be true. It has been more my experience that surgeons who exclusively practice the open or external approach are more critical and less accepting of the closed, or endonasal approach; and those of us who still use the endonasal approach more often accept that there is an alternative.

Personally, I use the endonasal approach in 85% of primary rhinoplasties and the external approach in the majority of revision cases. With proper planning in primary rhinoplasty, the external approach is rarely necessary. My personal indications for external rhinoplasty are in **Box 1**. However, in difficult cases, a transcolumellar incision can be added during endonasal rhinoplasty if closer inspection is required or difficulties arise that cannot be diagnosed or addressed by alar cartilage delivery.

Box 1
My indications for external rhinoplasty

- Extremely crooked nose, especially with complex septal curvature
- Lengthening a very short nose
- Significant deprojection and rotation of a very large nose
- Complex revision rhinoplasty

My personal indications for external rhinoplasty are: very crooked noses often require scoring with mattress sutures[12] as well as spreader and other grafts to stent the septum. Use of polydioxanone (PDS) flexible foil has been a big help in getting very crooked noses straighter, particularly when there is curvature of the caudal-most septum.[13] Rarely, extracorporeal septoplasty is used for complex septal deviation that requires an external approach.[14]

To lengthen a short nose, all 3 limbs of the tip tripod require lengthening. Centrally, a caudal septal extension graft is placed with spreader grafts and/or PDS flexible foil. The lateral crura also need to be elevated from the underlying mucosa and thrust downward. I find these maneuvers are best achieved through an external approach.

I have reduced very large overprojected noses through the endonasal approach, but in 2 patients within recent memory, I have needed to go back to get further reduction. So, for very large, overprojected noses, I also generally start with an external technique.

In revision rhinoplasty, unless the revision is only for minor irregularities or reductions, an external approach affords a better view of the distorted anatomy without further disturbance or distortion when delivering the lower lateral cartilages during an endonasal approach. When one or more prior surgeries have been performed, sutures and grafts may have been placed, structures may have twisted, and scar tissue has likely formed. Even if I obtain prior surgical notes, they may not be entirely accurate and will not reflect postoperative scarring and warping. Through an external approach, I can see better how form and function are compromised. During revision rhinoplasty, I often use multiple grafts placed in both anatomic and unanatomic areas that are made easier by the external approach.

One might invoke the same reasoning for why an external approach should be used for primary rhinoplasty as well. However, comprehensive knowledge of nasal anatomy, thorough examination, and solid understanding of the consequences of surgical maneuvers allows equivalent results with endonasal rhinoplasty. I have heard it argued that the external approach is better for teaching residents. But if all a resident sees is the external approach, they will never learn endonasal rhinoplasty. If it's about seeing, teaching, or understanding the anatomy better, then they should take one or more cadaver courses.

Quality rhinoplasty still takes years of study no matter what incision is used. It's akin to the revolution of endoscopic sinus surgery in the late 1980s and early 1990s. I was fortunate enough to have been trained in endonasal sinus surgery. The key to successful surgery was thorough knowledge of sinus anatomy and surgical landmarks. When endoscopic surgery was first introduced, complications skyrocketed to the point that endoscopic sinus surgery was the most common reason for otolaryngologists to be sued for malpractice.[15] Adding a telescope and getting a closer view of the sinuses did not automatically impart surgical knowledge. Individuals who might not otherwise have attempted advanced sinus surgery were emboldened by the false safety of a better view. Surgeons still need to take multiple courses with cadaver dissection and observe skilled teachers to become proficient at this procedure.

Minimally invasive surgery and minimizing incisions have become the mantra of many other surgical specialties.[16] There isn't one surgical specialty where you won't hear about smaller scars with quality results in both the medical literature and lay media. Why not learn how to offer the same choices to your rhinoplasty patients? When discussing the difference between endonasal and external rhinoplasty with prospective patients, I review the indications for my incisions. If they have seen or read about other surgeons who offered a different approach, I discuss that the incision is tiny and rarely visible, and avoid any denigration of another technique. If an external approach is chosen by the surgeon and the transcolumellar scar becomes visible at all, it would be likely only to someone who is up under their nose and close enough to be "counting nose hairs," However, it's still comforting to patients to be offered the opportunity to have an equally successful rhinoplasty without any external incisions and zero chance of visible scar.

Should the tip lobule be divided or preserved?

ADAMSON AND KIM

It is a rhinoplasty myth that if you divide the tip lobule you cannot preserve it. In fact, in many cases, division with reconstruction is much more preferable than preservation of a deformity. Therefore, we do not hesitate to use vertical lobule division (VLD) to correct tip abnormalities and irregularities, as it is a versatile and safe technique with predictable outcomes. We also distinguish between vertical arch division (VAD), which is a vertical division anywhere in the M-arch, and

VLD, which is vertical division within the lobule or domal arch. VLD can be used to decrease projection; to narrow a wide or boxy tip; to correct knuckling, bossae, tip asymmetry, or a hanging columella; and to improve rotation. It was first described by Goldman in 1957 for increasing tip projection and rotation endonasally.[12] It consisted of a vertical division of skin and cartilage lateral to the apex of the lobule and borrowing from the lower lateral cartilage to add length to the medial crus, or what is today known as the intermediate crus. Because the two anterior ends of the medial (intermediate) crura were sutured together, but were not resutured to the lateral crura, the division created instability and sometimes resulted in bossae, knuckling, asymmetries, and tip irregularities. Following this, cartilage excision techniques were introduced for vertical dome (lobule) division to correct deformities and/or shorten the lobular arch. Initially the cut cartilage ends were not secured to each other, but ultimately it was recognized that suturing the cut ends together increased stability and decreased longer term residual deformities. The next step in the development of VAD was incision only with overlapping and suturing the cartilage segments. This newer technique

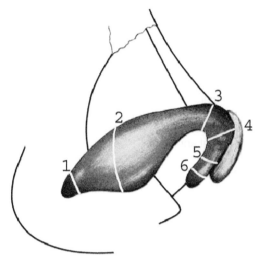

Fig. 2. Adamson and Kim. Vertical divisions of the M-arch. The various locations that have been described as sites to divide the M-arch: (1) hinge area, (2) lateral crural flap, (3) Goldman maneuver, (4) vertical lobule division, (5) Lipsett maneuver, and (6) medial crural feet.

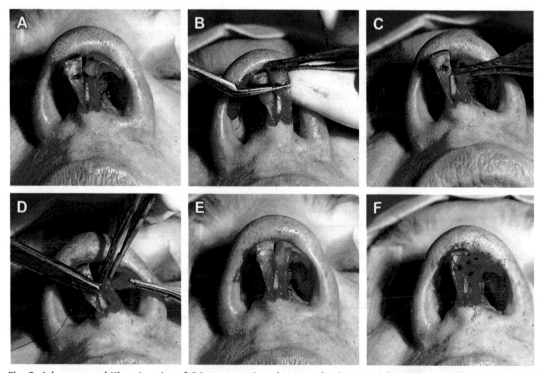

Fig. 3. Adamson and Kim. A series of 6 intraoperative photographs depicting the sequence of steps in vertical lobular division (VLD). (A) Site of the VLD shown marked. (B) Scissors shown cutting through lower lateral cartilage. (C) Overlapped cartilage ends. (D) Overlapped ends being sutured. (E) Pre-VLD basal view. (F) Post-VLD basal view (left side only).

was used to decrease the length of the lobular arch to decrease projection and/or improve lobular arch symmetry, at the same time increasing stability and decreasing revision rates.[13] In time, the versatility of this incision and overlap technique with suture stabilization has been applied to all regions of the medial, intermediate, and lateral crura.

The current terminology is to call these overlay techniques, and they can be performed wherever desired in the M-arch. So it can be seen that dividing the lobule has many applications and advantages. However, it is imperative to appreciate that "vertical division" does not necessarily refer to the Goldman technique uniquely.

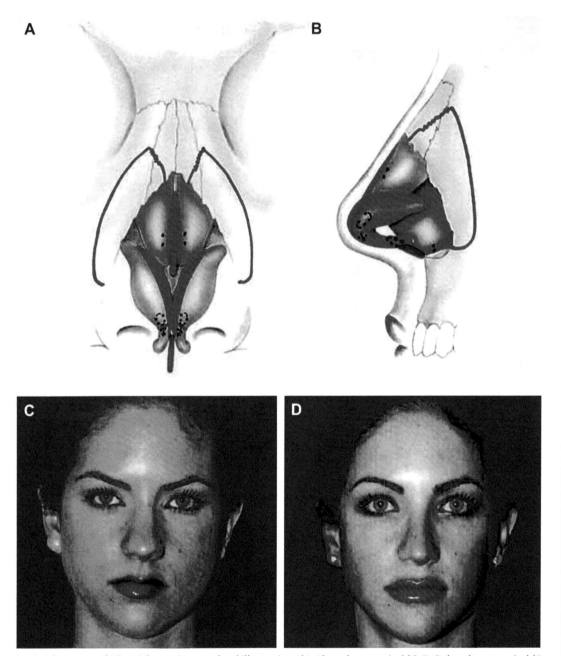

Fig. 4. Adamson and Kim. Schematic procedural illustrations (A, B), and presurgical (C, E, G, I) and postsurgical (D, F, H, J) patient photographs. Operative schematics (A, B) illustrating vertical lobule division and single-dome unit sutures for deprojection and lobule refinement. Frontal (C, D), right lateral (E, F), right oblique (G, H), and basal (I, J) views before and 30 months after rhinoplasty.

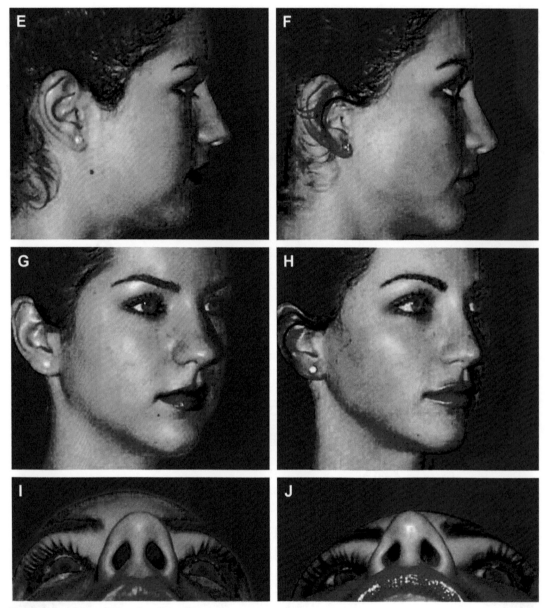

Fig. 4. Adamson and Kim. (*continued*)

Before dividing any cartilage, I make sure it is extensively released from the vestibular skin to allow for cartilage advancement. The location of the division determines the overall effect on the nasal tip: projection, definition, rotation, and nasal length (**Fig. 2**).[14] Division at the medial crural feet, followed by a medial crural overlay, will deproject and counter-rotate the tip and can be used to decrease excessive flaring of the medial crural footplate. Midmedial crus division can be used to adjust columellar asymmetries in addition to deprojection and counter-rotation with a medial crural overlay. Division at the junction of the medial and intermediate crus will result in tip deprojection, vertical shortening of the infratip lobule, and a diminished hanging infratip lobule or intermediate crura. At the dome or in the intermediate crus, division and overlap, or intermediate crural overlay (ICO), will deproject the tip and produce greater acuity of the domal arch and therefore lobular refinement. Asymmetric division, when needed, can improve lobule symmetry here with sutures concealed within the infratip. Division and overlay in the midlateral crus is a powerful maneuver for producing rotation and deprojection through a lateral crural overlay. When lobular contour is acceptable, division at the hinge area will depro-ject and rotate the tip. In all of these techniques, we reconstruct the M-arch with sutures to secure structural integrity and normal anatomy. The cut ends of cartilage are overlapped from 2 mm up to 6 mm in some cases and are secured with 6-0 nylon mattress sutures. One set of buried sutures is placed to set the length of the overlap. A second set of buried sutures is used to set the axis of the neo-arch. Alternatively, one can use 4-0 Vicryl su-tures in the lateral crus to fixate the cartilage seg-ments through the underlying vestibular skin. This can be used to overcome the technical challenge of burying sutures in this location (**Fig. 3**).[14] To avoid inflaring or collapse of the arch on contrac-tion of the skin–soft tissue envelope, overlapping suture fixation must be used.[15] Generally I use the cartilage segment closest to the lobule as the overlying segment.

Some may see the disadvantages of this approach as requiring increased operative time and disruption and weakening of the alar cartilages. While it may be a technically challenging technique,

use of an open approach facilitates proper execu-tion. Overlapping the alar cartilage gives the crus increased strength and support for the nasal tip. I find that it works best for the overprojected inferi-orly rotated tip because it results in either deprojec-tion, rotation, or both (**Fig. 4**).[14] It can be used to correct the M-arch length and asymmetry in addi-tion to irregularities of the lobular-columellar rela-tionship such as a hanging infratip. It can be tailored specifically to each side to achieve ideal shape and symmetry. It can be used to strengthen weakened, knuckled, or buckled cartilage. Alar notching is another concern raised by critics of VAD. The overlapping suture stabilization, how-ever, eliminates this and fortifies the arch.

Certainly each patient's individual anatomy should be taken into consideration, and VLD is not indicated in every case. Tip lobule preservation is indicated when vertical shortening is not needed and, for example, when rotation and projection are not an issue. These and other factors should be taken into consideration when planning an approach for each patient.

CONSTANTINIDES

The term "vertical dome division" was coined by Simons[6] to describe the cartilage division em-ployed in the Goldman tip technique in rhinoplasty. Adamson later expanded its use to include any maneuver that divides the alar cartilages along any point, calling it "vertical lobule division".[7] Mod-ifications of this term have been used by Lipsett to signify division across the medial crura. The distinction between vertical division, in which the tip cartilage is transected (usually preserving the underlying mucosa), with horizontal division, in which the tip lobular cartilages are left intact (intact strip) is important. Most rhinoplasties include hor-izontal division of the lateral crus, also known as cephalic trims. Both vertical and horizontal divi-sions can lead to cartilage instability and postop-erative knuckles or bossae. However, it is the vertical division that has created the most contro-versy, in particular in Goldman's and Simon's descriptions.

The Goldman tip was developed as a way to improve definition in New York City's ethnic rhino-plasty population by Irving Goldman in 1954. Simons, a Goldman pupil, further refined the oper-ation. In today's iteration, each alar cartilage is transected just lateral to the dome while preser-ving the underlying mucosa and then the medial crura are bound together, increasing projection and rotation while the lateral crura are allowed to fall away. A "hockey-stick" modification by

Simons alters the technique to include a medial cartilage excision in order to utilize the technique to decrease tip projection while still affecting rota-tion.[8] No attempt is made in either technique to restore the integrity of the alar cartilages; they are meant to be left discontinuous.

This purposeful lack of continuity of the alar car-tilages is what makes many rhinoplasty surgeons uncomfortable with this technique. Dr Simons' re-view article of his own experience reveals that he only uses it in less than 15% of his rhinoplasties (166 of 1271). All of his experience is with the en-donasal approach.[6]

Adamson, raised under Jack Anderson in the external approach, also transects the cartilages. However, he then restores the intact strip by over-lapping and then resuturing the transected carti-lages. Scoring, and more recently dome suture techniques, creates the desired tip definition, but with a smaller volume of cartilage overall. Adam-son's VLD is intended to decrease projection, much like the hockey-stick vertical dome division of Simons, but without leaving discontinuous car-tilages. This recreation of the intact strip theoreti-cally increases alar cartilage stability since the overlapping segment of cartilage doubles the cartilage thickness in the overlapped area. If increased projection is then required, standard techniques including lateral crural steal, medial crural advancement, or tip grafting is performed.

I worry about the Goldman tip. I worry that dividing the lateral crura from the medial crura leaves too much to chance during healing. If the difference in height between the new domes and the lateral crural remnant is too high, then unnatural shadows will occur lateral to the domes, creating a ball-like appearance to the tip. I worry that if the domes are sewn too tightly together in the midline, an uni-tip appearance may result as well, leaving a tent-pole appearance to the tip. Worse yet, if one medial crus is stronger or longer than the other, one dome will project excessively, creating an asymmetric tip and an overlong nostril on one side. These are not hysterical ruminations, but rather based on seeing such cases for revision in my own practice (**Fig. 5**).

On the other hand, I have had excellent experiences with Adamson's VLD. It takes Anderson's

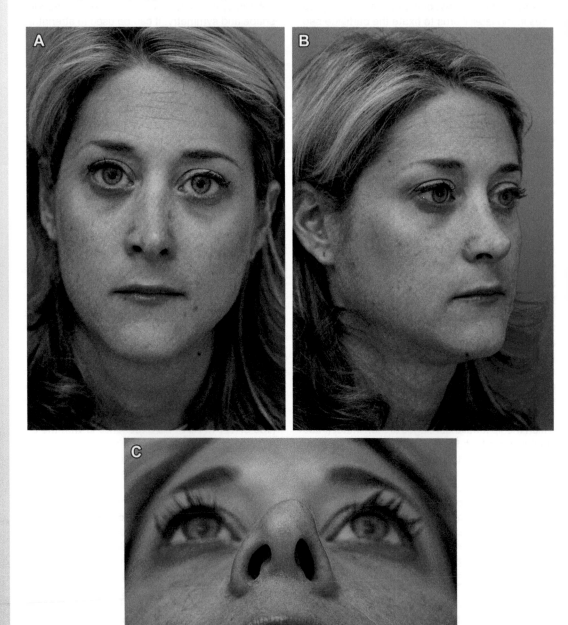

Fig. 5. Constantinides. (*A–C*) Asymmetric Goldman dome divisions resulted in marked projection of the left dome and an underprojected right dome, resulting in marked tip deformities in this thin-skinned revision patient.

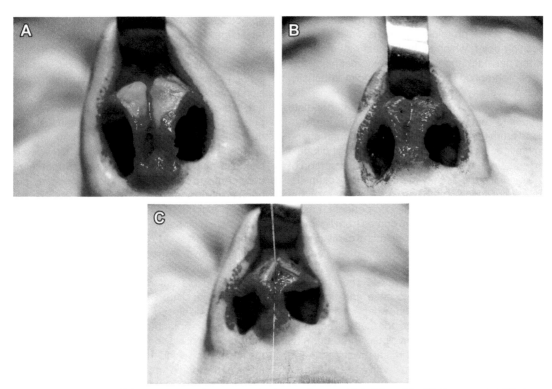

Fig. 6. Constantinides. (*A*) Overprojected, asymmetric alar cartilages with left knuckle. (*B*) Asymmetric VLDs have reduced projection while creating improved symmetry and restoring the intact strip. (*C*) Bilateral single-dome sutures and an interdomal suture create better domal definition.

tripod principle and applies it to central segments of the tripod. In a nose that is overprojected and long, vertical division at the domes with overlap and restoring the intact strip will create predictable rotation and shortening. In a nose that is overprojected and has neutral rotation, vertical division in the middle of the intermediate (middle) crus creates decreased projection while leaving rotation unchanged. In a tip with long, droopy medial crura, dividing them and overlapping them (eg, Lipsett) will straighten them and decrease projection (depending upon the amount of overlap). VLD increases the tools a surgeon has to effect precise lobular changes while strengthening the resultant construct (**Fig. 6**).

Goldman's tip technique, devised when rhinoplasty was in its infancy in the 1950s, is no longer required to overcome the broad ethnic noses with thick skin and weak cartilages. Indeed, using it in anyone without these characteristics requires

precise knowledge of what will happen in these noses over many years. If Dr Simons only performs it once in every 7 rhinoplasties, how many rhinoplasties (and years of follow-up) will it take a surgeon without his volume and experience to feel sure of when the technique does not increase risk of postoperative tip asymmetries and irregularities?

I see the Goldman tip as a technique that may remain useful in thick-skinned African American noses, in which the underlying cartilage framework will be difficult to see regardless of what is done intraoperatively. However, I prefer even in these noses to build rigid tip support with septal extensions, tongue-in-groove medial crural support, and strong tip grafts to increase projection and create as ideal a defined tip as these noses will allow. Goldman's tip cannot produce the amount of definition that structural grafting can in these challenging cases.

PEARLMAN

I will preface my answer with a "Yes, both." I try to preserve the tip lobule, but have no problem dividing the tip lobule when indicated.

The tip lobule is a complex, broad area that defines the apex of the nasal tip tripod and spans from the lateral to medial crura. The lateral crura intersect the intermediate crura at the dome. The dome's most prominent point is called the tip defining point, which is the highest external peak in the nasal tip and is seen as external highlights in photographs. The tip defining point is usually, but not always, at the cephalic edge of the dome. Further caudal-medially, the intermediate crura intersect with the medial crura. The intermediate crura are variable in length and impart shape to the lobule and infratip lobule. The infratip lobule extends from the domes to the cephalic portion of the medial crura as they merge into the columella. This entire intricate arch has variable shape, width, and strength for each of the components. Lastly, there are contributions to the domes from ligamentous attachments of the upper lateral cartilage and septal cartilage.

Rhinoplasty is not about following rote patterns, or one of a few preset formulas. The operation should address the specific nose and tip deformities present and change what is necessary with as little disturbance to the natural anatomy as possible. The more convoluted the deformity, the more complex the surgical treatment, and consequently, the more destructive of the natural anatomy. I attempt to preserve at least some portion of the tip lobule cartilage, especially in patients with thin skin. However, if the tip needs extensive changes in shape or projection, the lobule may need to be divided to obtain quality results (**Fig. 7**).

For a very wide tip in patients with medium or thick skin, the lower lateral cartilage can be divided at, or just lateral to, the dome. The classic dome division procedure is called the Goldman tip[17] and divides the vestibular skin as well. Simons[17] improved on this technique with the modified Goldman tip. The primary modification is a hockey-stick shaped cephalic trim of the lateral crura, preservation of the vestibular mucosa, and sewing the medial crura together below the actual peak of the resection. I have seen a number of rhinoplasty panels with photos of patients with nasal tip bossae, pinched tips, and otherwise deformed nasal tips being presented. Observations by either the presenter or panel often comment that it "must be from a Goldman tip or dome division." Usually it is not. I have seen many similar deformities in revision rhinoplasty patients, and far more often than not, the dome arch is found to be intact. My only personal caveat to *not* divide the domes is when the patient has very thin skin.

When the dome is broad, it can be narrowed by cephalic trim, dome sutures, scoring, morselization, cephalic "v-cut," or division. For many surgeons, all or some of these maneuvers are part of their algorithm for narrowing the nasal tip. Each maneuver has its benefit as well as its potential complications. My personal algorithm includes all of the above, in the order listed, excluding morselization. Morselization is unpredictable and can lead to variable deformity of the tip by irregular healing or buckling.

To reduce likely redundancy, Dr Peter Adamson, one of the co-contributors to this *Clinics in Facial Plastic Surgery*, described the "M-arch model" of the nasal tip.[18] He further refined VLD to 2 different areas of the lobule and will likely be discussing it in his answer. To summarize, dividing the arch at the dome treats a wide domal arch. Progressing more caudally, incising and overlapping the dome at the junction of the intermediate and medial crura can treat patients with broad flat tips and a plunging or hanging infratip lobule.

I was taught dome division over 25 years ago in selected patients as part of the "Mount Sinai" school of rhinoplasty as a resident under Dr William Lawson, and as a fellow with Dr William Friedman, and have had continued reminders over the years by Dr Robert Simons. As my practice matured, I would hear detractors speaking against dome division, and from time to time, I would cave in and stray from my teaching. I would narrow wide domes with cephalic resection and dome sutures (single or transdomal). Sometimes I added a "v-cut" at the apex of the dome to assist in narrowing. In occasional patients, sufficient narrowing still was not achieved, and I would need to go back and divide the domes to get further narrowing during revision surgery.

The only patients in whom I have reservation about dividing the domes, as well as other tip maneuvers including cephalic resection and dome sutures, is when patients have thin skin. Even in the latter cases, without dome division, I camouflage potential shrink-wrapping by an onlay of a tip "cushion" graft at the end of the procedure. These grafts can be paper-thin septal cartilage, crushed cartilage that was resected from one lateral crus, ear perichondrium, or temporalis fascia.

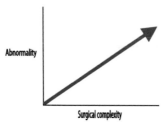

Complexity of rhinoplasty should mirror the surgical abnormality of the nose

Abnormality

Surgical complexity

Fig. 7. Pearlman. Graph depicting complexity of surgery with extent of abnormality to be addressed.

Surgery of the nasal tip is the most chal-lenging part of rhinoplasty. Nasal tip deformities are also the #1 reason patents seek revision rhi-noplasty.[10] Dividing the lobule is way down on the list of causes for tip deformities, and likely an uncommon cause in properly selected patients. At the risk of being redundant, it's more important to understand the variable anatomy, indications for each technique applied to the nasal tip, and the consequences of those techniques to reduce the incidence of complications.

Are alloplastic implants inferior to autologous implants?

ADAMSON AND KIM

Every implant has its advantages and disadvan-tages which must be taken into consideration when deciding which one to use. Currently there is no perfect implant material, but there are im-plants that are better than others depending on re-sources available and their intended use. The ideal implant should be readily available, inexpensive, easily carved and fixed to the recipient site without difficulty. It should not cause donor-site morbidity or lose volume and change shape over time. Prop-erties of the implant should match those of the recipient site in terms of rigidity and flexibility. If needed, the implant should be easily extractable without damage to the overlying skin–soft tissue envelope.[16] The ideal implant is inert and lacks contamination that may promote excessive inflam-matory reaction from the recipient site. It must be easily biointegrated by the host without excessive mesenchymal infiltration and capsule formation. The implant should not be carcinogenic or transmit infectious diseases. An ideal graft would be resis-tant to infection. It should not degrade into hazard-ous by-products nor act as a catalyst for autoimmune diseases.[17]

Implants can come from the patient as in auto-grafts, from other humans as in allografts or homo-grafts, from nonhuman species as in xenografts, or they can be synthetically manufactured as in allo-plasts.[18] I use the term "implant" to refer to any material placed in the nose for structural purposes while the term "graft" refers specifically to implants harvested from living sources. In my practice I most frequently use autologous cartilage due to its strength, structural support, versatility, and low rate of infection and resorption. These are some of the characteristics that have afforded it tremendous success in aesthetic and functional rhinoplasty.[19–21] Not only does it have the strength for structural support, but it can also correct subtle depressions and act as a filler for larger concav-ities. When used in children, preservation of the overlying perichondrium will allow for growth of the graft with the child. It can also be stored in deep postauricular pockets for use many years later without fear of resorption.[17]

Autologous cartilage can be obtained from the septum, conchal bowl, or rib. Septal cartilage, when available, lies within the same operative field, minimizing donor-site morbidity. It is preferred when straight grafts are needed. It can be har-vested via a hemi-transfixion, partial transfixion, total transfixion, or Killian incision. In open septorhi-noplasty, the interdomal ligaments between the medial crura can be divided for access. In revision cases where there may be scarring along the caudal septum, it may be advantageous to sepa-rate the ULCs from the dorsal septum. Hydrostatic dissection from injection of local anesthetic with epinephrine facilitates this procedure. Preservation of at least 1 cm of dorsal and caudal strut is neces-sary. Disarticulation of the dorsal septum from the ethmoid perpendicular plate must be avoided to prevent destabilization of the dorsum.

In revision cases where septal cartilage is not available, conchal cartilage is the next best alter-native with an acceptable level of donor-site morbidity. The curvilinear shape can easily dupli-cate the contours of the nasal skeleton. In addi-tion, the cartilage can be used with overlying skin for composite grafting. It is, however, limited by the quantity available for use, its relative weak-ness, and inherent shape. It can be harvested via an anterior or posterior approach with elevation of skin flaps through hydrodissection with a local anesthetic containing epinephrine. In the anterior approach, the skin is elevated in a subperichon-drial plane with care taken not to cross the antihe-lix or root of the helix. The posterior part of the cartilage is elevated in a supraperichondrial plane, leaving a thin layer of subcutaneous tissue on the graft which will enhance fixation in the recipient site. In the posterior approach, Colorado tip nee-dle cautery is used to elevate in the supraperi-chondrial plane to the external auditory meatus. The lateral aspect of the cartilage is elevated sub-perichondrially. A bolster dressing is applied post-operatively and secured with 3-0 nylon horizontal mattress sutures.

Costal cartilage can be used when multiple grafts or a large volume of grafting material, especially structural, is required. This may be the case with a multiply revised nose with a severe saddle deformity. In addition to warping, the main disadvantages of costal cartilage are the morbidities of postoperative pain, atelectasis, and potential pneumothorax. When harvesting costal cartilage, I prefer to use the right side to prevent the possibility of confounding cardiac chest pain. The patient is placed in the supine position so that the recipient site can be simultaneously prepared. Many surgeons prefer the 5th to 8th ribs and I usually use the 6th rib. Some may find that the 11th and 12th free-floating ribs are naturally straighter and require less carving and undergo less warping. A dorsal onlay graft can be fashioned using the osseous proximal one-third for stable bone to bone fixation to the nasal bones. This reduces warping by reducing the cartilage component of the graft. In addition, warping can be minimized by "balanced cross-sectional carving."[22,23] Placement of a K-wire centrally and longitudinally can also reduce warping.[24] The rib can be used for various other grafts such as premaxillary, caudal strut, alar battens, and tip onlay.

After an incision is made in the desired location, the overlying muscle is bluntly spread, not incised as to reduce postoperative pain. Perichondrium and periosteum are incised and elevated with a Freer, taking care to avoid the intercostal neurovascular bundle and the closely adherent pleura on the medial side. A malleable retractor is used to facilitate excision with a #10 blade. We frequently leave the inferior aspect of the rib intact, thereby reducing pain, splinting, and pneumothorax. It is important to remove the entire cortex and soak for 20 to 30 minutes in saline prior to sculpting. The pleura is examined for tears, the wound is irrigated with saline, and a Valsalva maneuver performed. If air bubbles are present, I would place a purse-string suture with a 4-0 Vicryl in the pleura around a red rubber catheter. The suture is then tightened and tied while the catheter is removed. If pneumothorax is still present, a chest tube is inserted and a postoperative chest x-ray is always obtained. Rib cartilage is my preferred graft when large quantities of cartilage are required. However, even with these maneuvers the main disadvantage of costal cartilage in my hands is postoperative warping.

Cranial bone grafts can be utilized for large saddle deformities of the dorsum. Membranous bone from the outer table of the parietal bone is preferred over endochondral grafts such as the iliac crest, due to its decreased risk of resorption. Donor-site complications include incisional alopecia, hematoma, infection, cerebrospinal fluid (CSF) leak, and intracranial bleeding. One commonly cited disadvantage is the thickness and rigidity which often results in edges that are difficult to sculpt and camouflage. When harvesting calvarial bone, a hemicoronal incision from the superior temporal line to the sagittal suture line overlying parietal bone is made. Elevation of the scalp proceeds in a subperiosteal plane and exposure is obtained with self-retaining retractors. The parietal bone provides the flattest bone. Care must be taken to avoid several boundaries such as the thin squamosa of the temporal bone which lies inferior to the superior temporal line. The superior sagittal sinus lies deep to the sagittal suture line and can result in exceptional bleeding if broached. The frontal sinus lies just anterior to the coronal suture line. Bone is harvested in a series of rectangular strips parallel to the sagittal plane in sections that are approximately 1.5 to 2 cm by 4 to 6 cm. A 4-mm otologic cutting bur is used to make a wide beveled trough. Dural tears and CSF leaks, should they occur, require a neurosurgical consult. A computed tomography scan of the head postoperatively rules out intracranial hematoma. The graft is prepared by ensuring all edges have been beveled and there are no sharp edges. Precise pockets must be made to stabilize onlay grafts. I tend not to use calvarial bone grafts today because in my experience with them they too frequently resorb.

Fascia can be harvested for use from the temple region from the superficial layer of the deep temporal fascia. Thickness ranges from 2 to 3 mm and they tend to maintain 80% of their thickness.[25,26] Another excellent source of fascia, especially if a posterior approach conchal cartilage graft is being taken, is mastoid periosteum, which is thinner than temporalis fascia.

Alloplasts have the advantage of unlimited availability, lack of donor-site morbidity, maintenance of shape and volume over time, and simplicity of placement. They have been successfully used by many surgeons for many applications, but the complications associated with them cannot be ignored. Implant instability in the nose, especially in the lower third, can lead to extrusion and damage to the skin–soft tissue envelope.[27] Due to the nature of its location on the face, the nose is an easily traumatized area. Trauma can affect the success of an alloplastic implant by making displacement and extrusion more likely to occur. Alloplasts should be used very cautiously in multiply revised noses as these patients frequently have loss of vascularity and a thin skin–soft tissue envelope, which can lead to increased likelihood of infection and/or extrusion. Alloplasts used to support the nose in, for example, a columellar strut, almost inevitably extrude due to the increased stress on the implant. We never use alloplasts for structural support. They should not be used in young males who engage in full-contact sports, due to the risk of trauma. Young individuals with alloplastic implants face a lifelong risk of extrusion which can occur decades after implantation.[17] In patients with a thicker skin–soft tissue envelope such as those of African and Asian descent, the risk of extrusion is somewhat less, but it still exists. For these patients and for patients who cannot accept donor-site morbidity, alloplasts are commonly used for dorsal augmentation due to the large amount of material that is required and the lack of donor-site morbidity. For these reasons I only ever consider an implant for dorsal augmentation, but never in the tip or for structural support.

Silicone implants are widely used in Asia for dorsal augmentation.[28,29] These have been successful because of the thicker skin–soft tissue envelope of Asian patients, which allows for greater cushioning and protection of the implant. The implant (Implantech, Ventura, CA) is commonly used in a prefabricated L shape as an onlay graft for the dorsum and tip as well as a premaxillary silicone implant. Series in Asia report acceptable rates of implant infection, extrusion, and malposition.[30] As the implant is nonporous, capsule formation occurs. However, micromotion between the implant and capsule does occur, which increases the risk of infection. Gore-Tex (W.L. Gore, Flagstaff, AZ) is a porous material which creates limited tissue infiltration due to the small average pore size of 22 μm.[31] This allows for implant stability with minimal tissue ingrowth and no capsule formation.[32,33] Infection and extrusion rates with Gore-Tex are less than those of silicone. It is more easily explanted than more porous materials such as mersilene. One should keep in mind that the complication rates with Gore-Tex are 4.5 times higher in revision than in primary rhinoplasties.[34] Nonetheless, having used mersilene mesh, Nylamid mesh (S Jackson Inc, Alexandria, VA), silicone, and Gore-Tex, my current preference is for Gore-Tex if autologous material is not preferentially available.

High-density porous polyethylene (HDPPE or Medpor; Porex Surgical Inc, College Park, GA) can provide more structural support than Gore-Tex due to its more rigid nature.[35] It should,

however, be used with caution, as any alloplast used to support the nose has an increased rate of extrusion. Medpor can be used when autogenous materials are not available or donor-site morbidity is unacceptable to the patient. This alloplast is easily carved and shaped into structures. In addition, it is available in preformed implants such as alar battens, L-strut, and total ULC and dorsal replacement. Extrusion rates are reported as 3.9% when used as onlays and support grafts.[35,36]

Rib cartilage allograft is available in abundant supply without the resultant donor-site morbidity of autogenous cartilage grafts. It consists of cadaveric bone from donors who have been screened for metastatic cancers and infectious diseases. Although animal studies initially raised concern about resorption, in practice it has been hypothesized that fibrous replacement may be maintaining the support needed for cosmetic rhinoplasty. It has been used successfully in the nose with acceptable rates of resorption and warping.[37,38] The warping seen with rib allograft is frequently a result of untreated graft infections and has been found to be less common than that seen with rib autografts.

Alloderm (LifeCell Corp, Branchburg, NJ) consists of cadaveric split-thickness skin grafts which have been stripped of dermal and epidermal elements to decrease antigenicity. Strict Food and Drug Administration manufacturing guidelines prevent transmission of infectious diseases. Once implanted, it is easily revascularized and remodeled into native tissues due to the blood vessels which are preserved in the allograft. It can be used to repair septal perforations and to camouflage sharp edges in thin-skinned individuals.[37] Initially Alloderm was felt to be relatively long lasting, but my experience is that resorption within a year or two coupled with its cost make it a less desirable implant.

For some surgeons, alloplasts are a reasonable alternative to autografts. However, I try to avoid using them due to the potential complications of infection, extrusion, and displacement. There is no perfect augmentation material, and any surgeon using a graft should take into consideration the limitations and potential complications of each type of graft or implant. Each of us also has our choice impacted by our own clinical experience.

CONSTANTINIDES

Surgeons have been searching for the perfect implant for centuries. Ivory, gold, wood, and stone have all been tried over the last 2000 years.

Only recently do we have a body of evidence supporting the use of alloplastic implants in rhinoplasty.

Some important studies regarding implants and their complications are listed under references at the end of this segment. For the most part, they show good safety and tissue tolerance, with an average of 3% to 9% complication rates.[9-11] So why doesn't everyone use them?

I began using expanded polytetrafluoroethylene (ePTFE) (Gore-Tex; W.L. Gore & Assoc, Inc, Flagstaff, AZ) as a fellow, and continued it for my first 10 years in practice. It was effective and well-tolerated in my first 25 private patients. When I heard from colleagues of problems, I was convinced that the problems came from a less rigorous implantation approach, inadequate implant preparation (I was impregnating the implant with antibiotic solution under negative pressure long before it became the company's standard protocol), or other controllable intraoperative scenarios.

I was starting to see some curious (aka troublesome) phenomena in some of my patients in the long term. In patients with thick skin, the implants had no issue. However, my practice was developing into a revision rhinoplasty practice so many patients were thin-skinned Caucasians with saddle noses. In these patients, I and my patients were seeing fine telangiectasias appear postoperatively in the dorsal skin over the implant that would not resolve with time. Furthermore, conservative treatments like needle cautery radiofrequency ablation and intense pulsed light therapy did not provide long-term improvement.

In the 1990s, I was also treating a number of patients with large septal perforations with saddling from cocaine abuse. I learned that in these patients dorsal onlays with ePTFE would gradually completely collapse, sinking into the nose gradually due to lack of L-strut support.

Finally, after about 5 years in practice, I started to see complications. My first is still among the worst. A diabetic man in whom I placed an ePTFE implant extruded the implant through the supratip skin. My second was an affluent banker whose implant twisted and hardened, resulting in a worse postop deformity than preop. My third was a teacher whose implant created a raging infection that threatened the viability of the dorsal skin. All of these complications occurred well after the rhinoplasty had been completed, ranging from 1 month to 1 year postoperatively.

As surgeons, we often make decisions based on rare but severe complications in our own practices. We cannot afford to wait for outcomes studies, valuable as they are, before changing our surgical practices. These three major complications, along with several more minor ones like smaller intranasal extrusions, prompted me to rethink the wisdom of alloplastic implants in the nose. Indeed, because of these my internal pendulum has swung completely away from alloplastic implants and to autologous. Now, I prefer septum, ear, or rib to ePTFE, porous polyethylene (MedPor; Stryker CMF, Newnan, GA), or silastic (although I continue to use silastic in the chin and cheeks). I will use cadaveric acellular dermis (AlloDerm; LifeCell Corp, Branchburg, NJ) only when a patient refuses temporalis fascia. For me, autologous trumps alloplastic every time … until the next new great implant is produced.

PEARLMAN

I will specifically address dorsal onlay grafts, since I never use alloplasts for any other grafts. Alloplasts have been described for columellar struts, spreader grafts, and alar strut grafts. Columellar strut grafts are in an area that is easily subjected to direct trauma. A blow to the tip of the nose with a stiff alloplastic graft can lead to displacement and/or extrusion. Spreader grafts and alar strut grafts have long surfaces adjacent to mucosa and, consequently, have more potential for contamination. Any mucosal tears during surgery could lead to bacterial colonization, or delayed exposure secondary to trauma. Dorsal onlay grafts are more isolated from rhinoplasty incisions, and don't have broad areas of contact with nasal mucosa.

For dorsal onlay grafts, it is important that a long, continuous graft is used. Unless the patient has very thick skin, small, piecemeal, or even flattened conchal cartilage grafts can warp or curl, and become visible. My first source for grafting material is the nasal septum. In both revision rhinoplasty and primary rhinoplasty, it is difficult to harvest a single septal graft long enough to span from the radix to the supratip. Until a few years ago, to obtain a long, straight graft, the choice would be between alloplasts or rib cartilage. Now we also have the option of diced cartilage in temporalis fascia (DCF).[19]

There are advantages and disadvantages to alloplastic implants. Alloplasts are easily obtained. They are simply taken off the shelf and implanted. There is no morbidity from obtaining them, and no shortage of supply. They are relatively easy to carve, and are readily available in a large number of anatomically correct shapes with nice smooth surfaces. Alloplasts are more commonly used in Asia, where rhinoplasty is more often an augmentation procedure. There is a very high success rate for alloplastic implants in Asia; this may be attributable to greater surgeon experience, or to the generally thicker skin in this patient population, which may be more protective of the implant. But trauma, even years later, can lead to infection and/or extrusion.

When choosing an alloplastic implant, I prefer ePTFE. It can be used as a preformed dorsal graft, or layered 1-mm and 2-mm patches. ePTFE has better tissue integration than silastic and therefore more resistance to future extrusion or delayed contamination. ePTFE has been used successfully with a reported infection rate ranging up to 2.6%[20] in larger series. Occasionally, some patients experience a tight contracted feeling around ePTFE implants. ePTFE should be avoided in patients with thin skin. I have seen the white color of the implant show through in such patients. Porous high-density polyethylene implants have had similar infection rates in earlier reports, but higher rates than ePTFE in a more recent study by Winkler and colleagues.[20] The other drawback to porous high-density polyethylene is that there is significant tissue ingrowth, and if there is a complication such as infection or displacement, it is very difficult to remove the implant.

One area where ePTFE is an excellent graft is in the radix. In a review of radix grafts, there were no complications when ePTFE was used and patients had visible or irregularities from cartilage grafts.[21] This success rate may be due in part to the remote placement of the ePTFE graft, away from mucosal surfaces and surgical incisions, and in part to placement of the implant in a tight pocket beneath the procerus muscle. I use this technique often in primary surgery on African American patients when all available septal cartilage is used for nasal strut and tip grafts. Use of the ePTFE precludes the need for harvesting conchal or rib cartilage for a primary rhinoplasty.

Over the past few years, I have shifted my dorsal graft of choice to a newer technique, DCF. It's not necessarily because this technique is superior to alloplasts, but it's natural, has a lower infection rate, and is more acceptable to patients. Prior to DCF, if alloplasts were eschewed, it would often be necessary to harvest autologous rib to get a long, straight dorsal graft. This adds time, morbidity, patient resistance, and a very small potential for pneumothorax. So I would often opt for an alloplastic implant, or at least offer patients the choice between autogenous rib and an alloplastic implant. Often, they would choose the alloplast given the low complication rate and ease of harvest (from a box).

Dorsal onlay with DCF can be performed with any cartilage, including septal or conchal remnants after other grafts are carved. Of course, rib can also be diced and rolled in temporalis fascia. I actually prefer using DCF to solid rib grafts in augmenting the nasal dorsum because of the smooth nature of the graft and lower potential for warping. Even in complex saddle nose reconstruction, extended spreader grafts are cantilevered to a broad caudal septal extension graft. A DCF graft is then placed on top of this structure to treat any remaining saddle deformity. Since shifting to DCF as my primary dorsal onlay for saddle nose deformity and becoming facile with harvesting temporalis fascia, I sometimes use folded or rolled temporalis fascia to obtain minimal dorsal or radix augmentation when needed.

One option that I did not discuss is irradiated cadaver costal cartilage grafts. Traditionally, these have been reported to have a high rate of resorption.[22] However, in a comprehensive, long-term study, Kridel and colleagues[23] reported a low 3.25% complication rate in 386 rhinoplasties. Dr Kridel has effectively revived an often ignored option for grafts in rhinoplasty. I have performed a few such procedures with success but don't have sufficient experience to qualify my personal opinion.

To summarize, I now use alloplasts only for radix grafts. The addition of DCF to my surgical repertoire has reduced my personal use of alloplasts for other applications. This does not, however, impart superiority, but rather a personal choice. Dr Kridel's study has also put cadaver costal cartilage grafts back on my list of surgical options.

Does release and reduction of the upper lateral cartilages from the nasal dorsal septum always require spreader graft placement to prevent mid one-third nasal pinching in reduction rhinoplasty?

ADAMSON AND KIM

Spreader grafts serve several functions in rhinoplasty, both functional and aesthetic. In performing rhinoplasty, it is important to consider their use once multiple support mechanisms of the ULCs have been compromised. I encourage liberal and what one might consider prophylactic use of internal nasal valve spreader grafts, as the adverse functional effects of a reductive rhinoplasty are often not seen until many years after surgery.

There are several ways that the support mechanisms of the ULCs can be compromised. The natural "T configuration" of the ULC with the dorsal septum is often disrupted by aggressive dorsal reduction. Resection of the dorsal septum, ULCs, and nasal valve apex mucosa results in severe ULC collapse. Creating submucoperichondrial junctional tunnels before hump reduction reduces scarring of the nasal valve apex and preserves the mucosal support for the ULC from the underside. I actually encourage dividing the ULC from the dorsal septum prior to hump reduction to allow a greater reduction of the dorsal septum as compared to the ULC and thereby attainment of the desired dorsal profile. When the height of the ULC is conserved, the natural T configuration of the nasal dorsum can be recreated. If the T-junction is resected, short nasal bones will not support the relatively longer ULCs. Aggressive rasping and misdirected osteotomies can result in complete disarticulation of the ULCs from the nasal bones at the keystone area. Aggressive cephalic trims and sacrifice of the scroll attachment of the ULC to the lateral crura may cause collapse of the free caudal border of the ULC and internal nasal valve obstruction. These are all situations in which support mechanisms of the ULCs have been compromised and are all cases in which internal nasal valve spreader grafts should be used.[39] In some cases, the ULC can be turned in to the dorsal septum as a turn-in flap, known as an auto-spreader. This may suffice in certain cases to provide the support needed otherwise from a spreader graft.

In addition to functional considerations, spreader grafts have important aesthetic applications. These include expanding width in an overly pinched dorsum, improving symmetry of the nose by filling in a concave dorsal line, straightening a twisted cartilaginous nasal dorsum when used as struts, supporting the tip if extended under the junction of the intermediate and lateral crura, lateralizing the lateral crura, lengthening the nose, or correcting a pinched tip deformity.

Spreader grafts are generally harvested from the most linear portion of donor cartilages, although curved grafts can be used to correct the direction of a twisted dorsum. They typically extend from the rhinion to the anterior septal angle. Extending them caudally can allow them to support a caudal extension graft and support the underside of the tip. They can also be extended cephalically to support collapsed nasal bones. I like to use grafts that are 1 to 4 mm in thickness, 3 to 5 mm in height, and 10 to 18 mm in length. If the goal is to preserve the width of the middle nasal vault, I use 1- to 2-mm wide grafts. If I need to expand a severely stenotic internal nasal valve angle, I use a wider graft of 2 to 4 mm fashioned from a double-layer septal or conchal cartilage graft. It should taper near the anterior septal angle to avoid excessive lateralization of the lateral crura, which can result in supratip fullness.

In an open approach, once the osteotomies have been completed, the skin–soft tissue envelope is retracted superiorly and the lower lateral crura are retracted inferiorly for exposure of the dorsum. Both spreader grafts can then be secured to the dorsal septum with 4-0 Vicryl horizontal mattress sutures. The ULCs are then attached on each side to the spreader graft complex with horizontal mattress sutures. Straightening the dorsal edge of the ULC by distracting its caudal end toward the anterior septal angle prior to suture placement is important when securing the ULCs. This prevents suturing buckled ULCs to the spreader graft complex. One should ascertain that the ULCs, spreader grafts, and dorsal septum are all engaged at the same depth with the suture to create a smooth dorsum.

In an endonasal approach the ULCs are not separated from the septum. Submucoperichondrial junctional tunnels should be fashioned. The spreader grafts are then placed in these tunnels. If wide mucoperichondrial flaps have already been elevated, the grafts can be secured to the apex of the dorsum using two transcutaneous stay sutures. I recommend a 4-0 Vicryl suture at each end of the spreader graft: one at the rhinion and the other at the nasal valve apex. Septal flaps are quilted, and the stay sutures are taped to the dorsum with Steri-strips for 1 week and then cut at the skin level.

Spreader grafts, especially when used in combination with flaring sutures, significantly increase the cross-sectional area of the internal nasal valve and increase nasal patency.[40] Rare complications include an excessively wide nasal dorsum and persistent nasal obstruction due to unaddressed nasal valve apex mucosal scarring. One must counsel patients with severe functional nasal valve obstruction that improved nasal breathing may only be achieved at the cost of a wider nasal dorsum. In short, we only use spreader grafts when necessary, but do not hesitate to use them if there is any concern regarding the long-term structural or aesthetic integrity of the dorsum.

CONSTANTINIDES

Like any surgical maneuver, how I use spreader grafts is based on the history of my training. I completed my fellowship with Dr Peter Adamson in 1994. At that time spreader grafts were just being recognized for their utility in preserving and, for some (including me), in improving the internal nasal valve. However, I and my mentor saw them at the time as a graft that was best used when the middle third was asymmetric. I used a spreader graft to support a collapsing ULC on one side when the septum deviated to the other side. Of course, when the middle vault was narrow bilaterally, I used them bilaterally.

With a high middle vault that required lowering, as in a tension nose, the same rule would apply. If after dorsal septal reduction the ULCs were too high, I trimmed them to the level of the dorsum after the osteotomies (since osteotomies might raise the height of the ULCs). If the dorsal septum was deviating to one side, a spreader graft was placed on the other. High dorsal deviations were difficult to correct, so the spreader graft allowed for camouflage of the deviation, creating a straighter appearance to the dorsal line. However, in a patient with a high middle third with no nasal obstruction, spreaders were placed only if the junction between the ULCs and the dorsal septum appeared too narrow. If the nasal bones at the K-region (where the ULCs and dorsal septum meets the nasal bones) were sufficiently wide, the ULCs did not require additional spreader graft support. If one nasal bone was long, occupying 50% of the middle third, then a spreader graft was placed on the other side to mimic the width. If both nasal bones were long, then no spreader graft was placed. I estimate that in high dorsa, I placed spreader grafts on one side or both in about 80% of these patients. This all changed 5 years ago.

In about 2006 I first heard of a technique where instead of trimming an excessively high ULC, one simply turned it in onto itself, creating an "auto-spreader flap" (**Fig. 8**).[12] Although not every ULC is a spreader flap candidate after dorsal reduction, often at least one side is. The more the dorsal septal reduction, the more excess ULC is available for this technique. In my strictly empiric experience, the technique not only adequately replaces

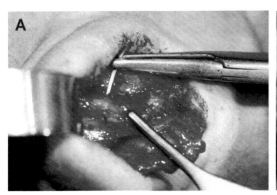
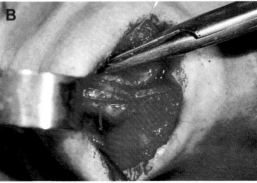
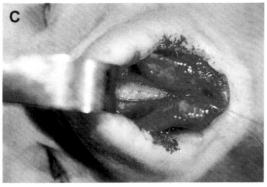

Fig. 8. Constantinides. Creation of an auto-spreader flap. (*A*) Horizontal bite through left ULC with 4-0 polydioxanone suture (PDS; Ethicon, Somerville, NJ). (*B*) The needle then passes through the septum, and then a horizontal bite is taken through the right ULC. (*C*) The resultant middle third is strong and the ULC-dorsal profile is smooth.

the need for spreader grafts in many cases, but it also improves the internal valve angle better that a spreader graft can. The additional advantage is that in a cartilage-deficient nose, no valuable cartilage is used on spreader grafts so more is available for other uses.

Now, I only use spreader grafts in reduction rhinoplasty when the ULC-dorsal junction is narrow *and* when the anatomy of the ULC does not allow for a spreader flap to be created. I do not reflexively put in spreader grafts in all noses, and I do not believe that the middle vault will eventually narrow over time so that it need be made excessively wide to begin with. In the absence of outcomes data that prove the opposite, I choose to believe instead that my own long-term results and happy patients are good evidence that my methods work well over time.

PEARLMAN

Rhinoplasty is an anatomically and aesthetically destructive operation. Excluding typical African American and Asian rhinoplasty, in the majority of cases, reduction is the primary goal. Reduction includes hump removal and lateral osteotomies to close an open roof. Once the nasal bones are brought inward, there is an associated, and possibly exaggerated, in-turning of the upper lateral cartilages. If you palpate the middle nasal vault on most noses, you can feel a step-off from the nasal bones to the ULCs. Close that any further, and you may risk both functional and aesthetic consequences. Narrowing the ULCs may compromise the internal nasal valve, creating functional nasal obstruction, and may also produce an aesthetic deformity.

Review of the literature confirms that lateral osteotomies narrow the middle vault and internal nasal valve.[24,25] This was confirmed in a study comparing different techniques for lateral osteotomies.[26] External perforating and internal continuous osteotomies both resulted in statistically significant reduction in the middle vault. The other invited authors for this issue of *Clinics in Facial*

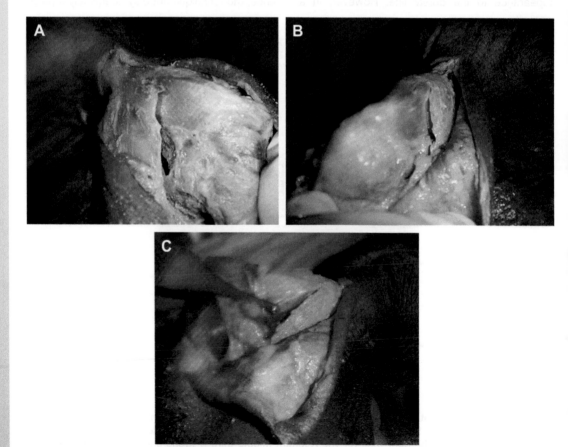

Fig. 9. Pearlman. Cadaver dissection of bony-cartilaginous junction.

Plastic Surgery have published on postoperative changes in the internal valve following lateral osteotomies, and will likely discuss this in more detail.

The ULCs do not insert end to end into the caudal nasal bones. The nasal bones overlap the cephalic end of the ULCs as a result of embryologic development. As a result of this relationship, the ULCs also don't necessarily continue in a straight line from the nasal bones. This step-off can be palpated in most noses (**Fig. 9**).

The cartilaginous dorsum is a single cartilaginous entity with the septum blending into the dorsal ULCs.[27] Cephalically, it is T shaped under the nasal bones, Y shaped at the rhinion, and I shaped near the septal angle. Reduction of the hump separates the septum from the ULCs, dividing them into 3 entities. Part of the horizontal portion of this structure is often removed as a dorsal hump is removed. This void is closed by lateral osteotomies, shifting the ULCs inward along with the nasal bones.

There are a number of aesthetic changes that can result from a narrow internal nasal valve. The most common is an "inverted V" deformity. Patients have a chevron-shaped shadow at the step-off from the nasal bones to the ULCs. Some patients portray this as a shadow, others describe a disconnection between the upper third and lower two-thirds of their noses. Another way patients describe this deformity are small "bumps" seen only on three-quarter views. Their primary nasal hump has been successfully reduced and is no longer visible on profile. This new or newly noticed postoperative bump is at the lateral bony-cartilaginous junctions.

As a resident, I was taught that these middle vault deformities were from overzealous rasping of the nasal bones and subsequent avulsion of the ULCs from the nasal bones. Subsequently the middle vault has been more carefully studied, and this narrowing is more likely from the relationship of the ULCs with the nasal bones and how they either change or narrow in parallel given the shape of this attachment. This has also been refuted in rhinoplasty texts.[28] If these lateral "bumps" are merely rasped further, it just moves

---

Box 2
Indications for spreader grafts in primary rhinoplasty

1. Reduction of a large nasal hump
2. Narrowing of wide nasal bones
3. Short nasal bones
4. Tension nose
5. Visibly narrow middle vault with palpable step-off from nasal bones
6. High osteotomies

---

the junction superiorly, since the cause isn't out-turning of the caudal nasal bones but a concave step-off to the ULCs.

The answer to reducing the incidence of middle vault deformities is to support the ULCs during rhinoplasty. The most commonly used technique is placing spreader grafts. They aren't necessary in every rhinoplasty, but in my opinion are necessary in a majority of reduction rhinoplasties. My indications for using spreader grafts in primary rhinoplasty are in **Box 2**. After considering these indications, I find that I am using spreader grafts in over 90% of my primary rhinoplasties.

There are numerous techniques for placing spreader grafts in rhinoplasty. They can easily be inserted during endonasal as well as external rhinoplasty. Endonasal techniques may include a precise pocket, suture, or tissue glue fixation.[29] To the uninitiated, it may seem easier to place spreader grafts through an external approach, but with practice, spreader grafts can be performed through either approach with consistent success.

When looking back at what I considered good results a decade ago, when I was only using spreader grafts for revision rhinoplasty, I can see some shadowing along the middle vault in a number of my rhinoplasty patients. Most of these patients were happy with their results, but looking back, I feel the results are not acceptable by today's standards.

Analysis: over the past 5 years, how has your technique or approach evolved or what is the most important thing you've learned in doing rhinoplasty?

ADAMSON AND KIM

One of the changes in my approach to rhinoplasty can be seen in the consultation process. Although

I have always asked the prospective patient to "tell me a little bit about your nose," now I also like to specifically ask them how long they have been thinking about having the procedure and what has been holding them back from having the procedure. This often reveals very specific concerns or fears that I can address. This helps the patient identify specifically what bridges need to be crossed before they can make a positive decision to proceed, and also helps me to identify who may be a poor candidate because of unrealistic fears that cannot be assuaged. With a patient population that increasingly seems to expect perfection and for accountability to lie solely with the surgeon, I am very specific about asking the patient how their objective rhinoplasty results will actually change their quality of life. This is a significant indicator as to whether a patient will be satisfied or not and whether he or she will be a good candidate.

For many years I relied upon the very utilitarian tripod concept of Anderson for my analysis and tactical planning for nasal tip dynamics. However, since introducing the M-arch model I have used this exclusively. It has expanded my theoretical thinking and tactical options and has been a very reliable tool to increase the quality and consistency of my nasal tip outcomes.

In considering surgical techniques, I generally prefer the open approach as I have for many years, but today undermine only as much as necessary. Thin-skinned patients who may have minimal dorsal reduction or tip refinement have very minimal undermining of the anterior portion of the lobule and nasal bridge, whereas patients who may have larger dorsal or tip reductions required or have very thick skin require more extensive undermining for better redrapage.

I recently reviewed the frequency of use of tip contouring techniques in my practice in a paper, "Evolution in Nasal Tip Contouring Techniques: A 10-Year Evaluation and Analysis." I found a significant reduction in tip reductive maneuvers and a significant increase in tip stabilizing and strengthening maneuvers. Specifically, medial crural excision, lobule scoring, lateral crural release, and cephalic trim were not being performed as often in later cases while there was an increase in lower lateral crural strut grafts, alar margin grafts, lateral crural overlay, columellar plumping grafts, and supratip grafts. While cartilage excisional techniques decreased over time, there was no change in soft tissue excisional techniques and an increase in stabilizing and strengthening techniques. I noted that this evolution of rhinoplasty techniques was also associated with a reduction in revision rates, although this finding was not found to be statistically significant.[41]

Cartilage arch

I have always extolled the virtues of leaving a very strong cartilaginous M-arch, and over the last 5 years, more than ever, leave a minimum of 8 mm, and frequently leave even 10 mm of lower lateral crural width. I have found it critically important to analyze the strength and contour of the cartilage arch in making the decision as to how much excision there should or should not be, rather than strictly referring to a numeric. Occasionally I will incise the cephalic margin and allow it to "turn-down" so that it decreases the bulk of the lateral supratip but still confirms some strength to the scroll region. Although I have utilized cephalic margin turn under flaps to increase the strength of the cephalic lower lateral crural margin, in general I have found that with a minimal cephalic incision the width of this cartilage is insufficient to have any significant strengthening impact on the residual lower lateral cartilage cephalic margin. And so in these cases I am more likely to resort to a lateral crural mini-strut graft if there is a convex or concave deformity or a full lateral crural strut graft if there is an associated functional deficit with collapsing of the lower lateral crus.

I am still a strong advocate of VLD, emphasizing as always that this does not refer to the Goldman technique, per se, but refers to any vertical division in the M-arch. Specifically, I am using the lateral crural overlay technique more frequently, especially in cases where I wish to obtain more rotation and deprojection. Differing from some other authors, I prefer to suture the overlay with a through-and-through suture of 4-0 Vicryl which passes through both sections of the overlay and cartilage in addition the vestibular skin, with the knot being tied in the vestibule. A mini Keith needle is used to secure the ideal degree of overlap, making this suture easy to place. It is necessary to be sure that in doing so, the vestibular skin is drawn inferiorly adequately so that with ultimate closure of the marginal incision there is no tendency for alar margin retraction. In cases where a lateral crural strut graft is also going to be placed, the indications being mentioned above, I do suture the overlying cartilage edges of the lateral crus first, place the lateral crural strut graft, and then transfix the lateral crural overlay and the lateral crural strut graft and the vestibular skin with one transfixion suture, as noted above.

In cases of more severe cephalic malposition of the lower lateral cartilages, it is necessary to completely free up the hinge area of the lower lateral cartilage, place an extended lateral strut graft of about 25 mm, and replace the hinge or foot of the lateral crus in a more inferior pocket. Because I frequently found it difficult to obtain strong enough or long enough cartilage from the septum, and did not always feel that this specific maneuver demanded a rib graft, I have resorted to placing lateral crural strut grafts about 20 mm in length in order to flatten and overall improve the apparent malposition of such cartilages. This can be reasonably accomplished in the majority of cases.

Nasal tip contour

As tip suturing techniques became more finessed, I, along with most surgeons, moved away from lobule scoring to achieve ideal tip contours. However, I have gone back to using light scoring techniques in patients with moderate to thicker lobule cartilage so that I may create the ideal lobule aesthetic and then stabilize this with single-dome unit or double dome unit sutures. I believe this gives a greater degree of exactness in refinement. Although I still use double dome unit sutures, unless these are very accurately placed they can sometimes introduce deformities into the lobule. And so in general I have come to prefer single-dome unit sutures followed by an interdomal suture to stabilize the domal complexes bilaterally.

I tend to use fewer tip grafts now than in earlier days, specifically the infratip lobular or shield graft. When doing so, or in fact when placing almost any lobular graft, I am assiduous about feathering the cartilage as I always was, but now in almost all cases I will camouflage the graft with soft tissue sewn into place. I most frequently obtain this soft tissue from between the intermediate and medial crura on the initial approach to the caudal septum. I am using more nasolabial angle grafts, preferably a single portion of cartilage which is sutured into place at the posterior columella, to obtain final refinements to increase rotation at the end of the procedure where indicated.

Dorsal augmentation

With regard to the nasal dorsum, today even if I am only effecting a moderate reduction I am much more aggressive in assessing the rhinion and the need for a spreader graft. I have come to realize that with time and scar contraction it is not infrequent that there is the creation of a small divot or depression in the rhinion region with collapsing of the medial and cephalic aspects of the ULC. In minimal dorsal reductions I will frequently suture the medial aspects of the ULCs, either in association with an auto-spreader or with a true spreader graft, to maintain integrity in this region for the long term. I do use auto-spreaders occasionally, but in my experience they are not always especially effective as they are frequently too weak or irregular to do the job that is required. As mentioned, they may be most effective at the rhinion, but if there is any question about their efficacy in the middle third I will place a true spreader graft.

Regarding radix grafts, I will use them when necessary but will not look for a reason to use them. In my experience, even those radix grafts that are shaped and feathered in detail and are secured with percutaneous transfixion sutures too frequently leave slight palpable irregularities that are not satisfactory for the patient. These most commonly occur at the rhinion/radix graft junction. This is true primarily for thin and moderately skinned patients. Today if grafting is required here I prefer to place soft tissue, either intercrural as described above, or mastoid or temporalis fascia.

I have moved to using rib grafts for dorsal augmentation more frequently than ePTFE (Gore-Tex), but find as many others have that there can still be issues with graft warping in spite of the best measures to prevent this. From my perspective the ideal dorsal augmentation material has yet to reveal itself.

Alar base reduction

Finally, I have long been a proponent of alar base reduction. Notwithstanding this, I feel that with globalization there is indeed a changing perception of beauty. One of the aesthetic components of this is that the nasal base can be somewhat wider than in the previously idealized narrow Caucasian base. I therefore perform alar base reductions more conservatively and in fewer cases than in previous years. During the 1950s we saw noses that were more rotated with narrower and more sculpted tips. In more recent times, a comparatively wider dorsum and fuller tip is preferred by many patients.[42] Many attractive people today have a lobule that is somewhat wider than we have seen in the past. Compared to several years ago, I find that I am performing fewer alar base reductions, taking down less of the dorsum, reducing minimally, and taking precautions to prevent overly narrowing the lobule. Less is more in this day and age. Tailoring surgery to each patient's individual needs and aesthetic ideals is crucial to a successful result, a goal which remains our constant challenge.

CONSTANTINIDES

I finished my fellowship with Dr Peter Adamson in Toronto, Ontario in 1994, so I have just completed nearly 20 years in clinical practice performing from 100 to 200 rhinoplasties per year. The past 5 years, or about the latest one-third of my career, has been a time for nuanced implementation of new maneuvers to see if they work better than older ones. Rhinoplasty basic concepts have been solidly in place with few changes during this time. For example, the order that I perform my surgical steps (open the nose–septum–dorsal reduction–osteotomies–middle third work–tip work) has not changed since my fellowship. How I perform each basic step saw some changes in the first 5 to 10 years in practice. For example, I changed from rasping to a dorsal osteotomy in the first 5 years in practice, reserving rasping for small changes or smoothening only. I changed from a running continuous osteotomy to a perforating intranasal osteotomy after about 7 years in practice.[13] The basic ways that I achieve reductions in nasal length, projection, and rotation have not changed much over the past 10 years, incorporating vertical lobule division frequently.[14] My technique for alar base reduction has not changed since fellowship.[15]

Over the past 5 years what has changed is how I approach dorsal augmentation, how I use tip grafts, my philosophy toward alloplasts, how frequently I use rib grafting, and how I manage complex septal deviations. For dorsal augmentation I now rely exclusively on diced cartilage wrapped with temporalis fascia (DCTF graft) (**Fig. 10**). I use Rollin Daniel's techniques and have found that Alloderm works as well as temporalis fascia while Surgicel does not.[16] For larger augmentations I now use rib cartilage, preferring autogenous over donor rib grafts. Even when I use rib grafting, though, I still use the DCTF graft as a final out layer over the rib construct. It provides softer contours, camouflages irregularities, and creates more natural transitions between the dorsal graft and the side walls.

I no longer use large Sheen tip grafts to increase tip projection. I have reverted entirely to a sequence of incremental projection:

1. First I create a strong base with a septal extension graft.
2. Then I free the medial crural feet completely from all septal ligamentous attachments.
3. I then advance the medial crura onto the septal extension graft using a tongue-in-groove technique.
4. I create domal definition and further projection with single-dome and interdomal sutures.

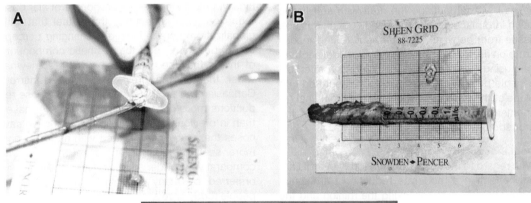

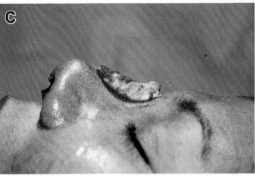

Fig. 10. Constantinides. Creating a diced cartilage temporalis fascia (DCTF) graft. (*A*) Cartilage is finely diced with a #15 blade, then packed into a 1-mL syringe. (*B*) Temporalis fascia is sewn around the outside of the syringe. (*C*) The DCTF graft is ready for implantation.

A

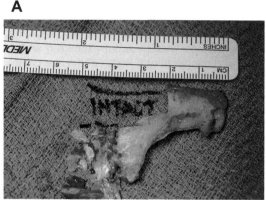

B

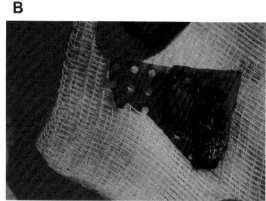

Fig. 11. Constantinides. (*A*) Excised septal cartilage and bone, indicating an intact superoposterior area where septal cartilage is left attached to perpendicular plate of ethmoid in situ. (*B*) Perforated PDS Flexible Plate 0.15-mm thick construct rebuilds a straight septum during the extracorporeal septoplasty. This is then inserted and secured end to end with the intact superoposterior septal cartilage and to the ULCs. Spreader grafts or auto-spreader flaps are used to help support the middle third (not shown).

5. Finally I will use a small infratip lobule graft or Peck grafts to achieve final projection and rotation.
6. I use crushed cartilage or cephalic trim grafts to transition from the tip graft laterally so the entire complex flows from tip to ala with strong, smooth lines.[17]

My philosophy toward alloplasts has been discussed in detail with my answer to the earlier discussion: *Are alloplastic implants inferior to autologous implants?*

Rib grafting has become a bigger part of my practice over the past 5 years. Although I still use ear cartilage for many revision problems, I now use rib grafting when I require strong lateral sidewall support in the form of batten grafts or lateral crural strut grafts. However, I believe that septal cartilage, when available, is still the best material for these grafts. I also of course use rib for large dorsal augmentations when dorsal strength has been weakened, either from over-resection of the L-strut or large septal perforations. However, when the dorsum is strong but over-resected creating a saddle, the DCTF graft is often adequate and ear can be used instead of rib.

Complex septal deviations that create dorsal deviations were handled by me for 15 years by an aggressive septoplasty followed by camouflage techniques to create straighter dorsal lines. For example, a deviation of the dorsal L-strut to the right might be improved by placing 1 or 2 thick spreader grafts on the left, camouflaging the deviation. However, these techniques always left me with less than ideal results. Some surgeons had started removing the entire L-strut and then reconstructing it with rib grafting. This seemed a little like throwing the baby out with the bath water to me, an overaggressive effort with a great cost to patient recovery and surgical effort. When I heard Wolfgang Gubisch speaking about extracorporeal septoplasty, I was intrigued with the possibilities.[18] However, I was afraid that the rebuilt septum would not be strong enough and that I would trade a crooked L-strut with a saddle.

Last year, the introduction of the PDS Flexible Plate (Ethicon, Inc, Somerville, NJ) allowed me for the first time to effectively perform extracorporeal septoplasty with acceptable risks to dorsal contour. My early experience with this material for complex septoplasty has left me excited that for the first time I can create truly straight L-struts in very deviated noses without the need for rib harvest (**Fig. 11**). I have been cautiously using it for complex septoplasties with excellent outcomes to date. However, I am also cautious not to become beguiled by a new product without strong clinical evidence of effectiveness over time. Fortunately, the European experience and Miriam Boenicsh's work has gone a long way to assuage my early doubts.[19] As in all things rhinoplasty, time will tell if this material will live up to its early promise.

PEARLMAN

Rhinoplasty has long been referred to as an art (Tardy). However, I feel that successful rhinoplasty is more analogous to architecture. Art involves creativity, skillful hands, and an aesthetic eye. Architecture is more about understanding construction, structure, support, and their relationship to the surrounding environment. An artist applies paint to a page, chips away at stone, or molds clay to create a concrete aesthetic image. An architect uses their understanding of structure and the strength of their materials to create a functional yet visually pleasing composition. The Modernist and Bauhaus movements revolutionized architecture, as I feel structural grafting revolutionized rhinoplasty.

Rhinoplasty was once a purely reductive procedure. The profile and nasal tip were reduced to the smallest or lowest existing point on the nasal profile to obtain a balanced result. Now, we are creating stronger noses with more attention to natural appearances and the maintenance of function. In keeping with the notion that "form follows function," spreader grafts were once used mostly in revision rhinoplasty, to restore middle vault patency. From past experience and careful scrutiny of the results of reductive rhinoplasty, spreader grafts are now commonly used in primary rhinoplasty to maintain middle vault function and improve aesthetics. Spreader grafts also serve to bridge the bony vault to the nasal tip, and smooth out the gentle curve that begins at the brow and ends at the nasal tip. This is the brow-tip curve that we were taught as residents, only now it's smoother.

Moving down to the lower one-third of the nose, I would like to credit Dr Dean Toriumi in what I feel was a landmark publication on rhinoplasty in 2006.[7] The diagram on the cover of that issue of *Archives in Facial Plastic Surgery* had topographic lines demonstrating a gentle curve of the tip to the ala and a convexity then concavity ascending from the alar rim delineating the alar crease. I often review these curves with revision rhinoplasty patients as well as primary rhinoplasty patients who have naturally deep alar creases. Another way to visualize these curves is by looking at nasal shadows and highlights. Abnormal highlights require reduction and abnormal shadows indicate the need for grafts.

Strength and position of the alar cartilage are both important for the nasal tip. Any weakness in alar support requires grafting to assure that tip reduction doesn't further compromise form and function of the external nasal valve. Lately, I have become more vigilant about examining and discussing the depth and length of the alar creases, especially in revision rhinoplasty. Weakened alar support results in deep alar creases that extend to the alar rims. Causes for alar weakness are cephalic orientation of the lateral crura, and weak or concave lateral crura.

Aesthetically, in patients who have weak alar support, their nostrils may appear almost "stuck on." This is much more commonly seen in revision rhinoplasty patients. This disconnect is often hard for patients to verbalize other than "not liking" the shape of the tip of their nose. They may say their tip is too wide, when it's really this separation of nostril from the tip. Evaluation is aided by reviewing all photographic views including the submental view. Weak ala can be seen by bowing in or insertion below the tip of the nose. Initially, patients protest the suggestion that grafts be added when they feel they already have wide nasal tips. Elevating the alar rim with an applicator or blending out shadows during computer imaging helps to demonstrate how grafting will actually make the tip appear more natural, and even smaller. There are a number of options for restoring alar rim support. These include alar strut grafts, alar batten grafts, cephalic turn-in grafts,[30] and rim grafts.[31]

Rhinoplasty has evolved rapidly over the past few decades, more than any other procedure in facial plastic surgery. Paradigm shifts such as deep plane dissection, fat transfer, transconjunctival approaches, and fat repositioning occur in facelift, blepharoplasty, browlift, and even resurfacing every 10 to 15 years. In rhinoplasty, such shifts occur almost from year to year. Tastes in what patients are seeking also change over time. Patients and surgeons appear to be more discerning, and even demanding, regarding the results of rhinoplasty. Most patients today seek refined, natural, and ethnically suitable results.

ACKNOWLEDGMENTS

Dr Steven Pearlman would like to thank Dara Liotta, MD for article editing.

REFERENCES: ADAMSON & KIM

1. Dayan S, Kanodia R. Has the pendulum swung too far?: trends in the teaching of endonasal rhinoplasty. Arch Facial Plast Surg 2009;11(6):414–6.

2. Zijlker TD, Adamson PA. Open structure rhinoplasty. Clin Otolaryngol 1993;18:125–34.

3. Vuyk HD, Olde Kalter P. Open septorhinoplasty: experiences in 200 patients. Rhinology 1993;31:175–82.

4. Adamson PA, Smith O, Tropper GJ. Incision and scar analysis in open (external) rhinoplasty. Arch Otolaryngol Head Neck Surg 1990;116:671–5.

5. Toriumi DM, Mueller RA, Grosch T, et al. Vascular anatomy of the nose and the external rhinoplasty approach. Arch Otolaryngol Head Neck Surg 1996;122(1):24–34.

6. Adamson PA, Litner J. Open rhinoplasty. In: Papel ID, editor. Facial plastic and reconstructive surgery. 3rd edition. New York: Thieme; 2009. p. 529–46.

7. Adamson PA. Open rhinoplasty. Otolaryngol Clin North Am 1987;20:837–52.

8. Gunter JP. The merits of the open approach in rhinoplasty. Plast Reconstr Surg 1997;99:863–7.

9. Kamer FM, McQuown SA. Revision rhinoplasty: analysis and treatment. Arch Otolaryngol Head Neck Surg 1988;114:257–66.

10. Bagal AA, Adamson PA. Revision rhinoplasty. Facial Plast Surg 2002;18:233–44.

11. Adamson PA, Doud Galli SK. Rhinoplasty approaches: current state of the art. Arch Facial Plast Surg 2005;7(1):32–7.

12. Goldman IB. Panel: questions and answers on rhinoplasty. Eye Ear Nose Throat Mon 1957;36(8):476–7.

13. Funk E, Chauhan N, Adamson PA. Refining vertical lobule division in open septorhinoplasty. Arch Facial Plast Surg 2009;11(2):120–5.

14. Adamson PA, Litner J, Dahiya R. The M-Arch Model—a new concept of nasal tip dynamics. Arch Facial Plast Surg 2006;8(1):16–25.

15. Adamson PA, McGraw-Wall BL, Morrow TA, et al. Vertical dome division in open rhinoplasty: an update on indications, techniques, and results. Arch Otolaryngol Head Neck Surg 1994;120(4):373–80.

16. Costantino PD, Freedman CD. Soft tissue augmentation and replacement in the head and neck: general considerations. Otolaryngol Clin North Am 1994;27:1–12.

17. Adamson PA, Ansari K. Grafts and implants in rhinoplasty—techniques and long term results. Operative Techniques in Otolaryngology-Head and Neck Surgery 2008;19(1):42–58 Friedman C, editor. Elsevier.

18. Vuyk HD, Adamson PA. Biomaterials in rhinoplasty. Clin Otolaryngol 1998;23:209–17.

19. Tardy ME, Denny J, Fritsch MH. The versatile cartilage autograft in reconstruction of the nose and face. Laryngoscope 1985;95:523–33.

20. Sheen JH. Secondary rhinoplasty. In: MacCarthy JG, editor. Plastic surgery. Vol 3, the face, part II. Philadelphia: W. B. Sauders Co; 1990. p. 1895–923.

21. Ortiz-Monasterio F, Olmedo A, Oscoy LO. The use of cartilage grafts in primary aesthetic rhinoplasty. Plast Reconstr Surg 1981;67:597–605.

22. Gibson T, Davis WB. The distortion of autogenous cartilage grafts: its cause and prevention. Br J Plast Surg 1958;10:257–73.

23. Adams WP, Rohrich RJ, Gunter JP, et al. The rate of warping in irradiated and nonirradiated homograft rib cartilage: a controlled comparison and clinical implications. Plast Reconstr Surg 1999;103:265–70.

24. Gunter JP, Clark CP, Friedman RM. Internal stabilization of autogenous rib cartilage grafts in rhinoplasty: a barrier to cartilage warping. Plast Reconstr Surg 1997;100(1):161–9.

25. Cheney MC. Auricular reconstruction. In: Fewkes JC, Cheney MC, Pollack SV, editors. Cutaneous surgery. Boston (MA): Lippincott; p. 33.1–33.16.

26. Miller PA. Temporalis fascia graft for facial and nasal contour augmentation. Plast Reconstr Surg 1988;81:523–33.

27. Berghaus A, Stelter K. Alloplastic materials in rhinoplasty. Curr Opin Otolaryngol Head Neck Surg 2006;14(4):270–7.

28. Shirakabe Y, Suzuki Y, Lam SM. A systematic approach to rhinoplasty of the Japanese nose: a thirty-year experience. Aesthetic Plast Surg 2003;27:221–31.

29. Yang J, Wang X, Zeng Y, et al. Biomechanics in augmentation rhinoplasty. J Med Eng Technol 2005;29:14–7.

30. Tham C, Lai YL, Weng CJ, et al. Silicone augmentation rhinoplasty in an Oriental population. Ann Plast Surg 2005;54(1):1–5.

31. Schoenrock LD, Reppucci AD. Correction of subcutaneous facial defects using Goretex. Facial Plast Surg Clin North Am 1994;2:373–88.

32. Maas CS, Gnepp DR, Bumpous J. Soft-tissue response to synthetic biomaterials. Otolaryngol Clin North Am 1994;27:195–201.

33. Berman M, Pearce WJ, Tinnon M. The use of Gore-tex E-PTFE bonded to silicone rubber as an alloplastic implant material. Laryngoscope 1986;96:480–3.

34. Godin MS, Waldman SR, Johnson CM Jr. Nasal augmentation using Gore-Tex. A 10-year experience. Arch Facial Plast Surg 1999;1(2):119–21.

35. Romo T, Sclafani A, Sabini P. Use of porous high-density polyethylene in revision rhinoplasty and in the platyrrhine nose. Aesthetic Plast Surg 1998;22:211–21.

36. Romo T 3rd, Kwak ES, Sclafani AP. Revision rhinoplasty using porous high-density polyethylene implants to reestablish ethnic identity. Aesthetic Plast Surg 2006;30(6):679–84 [discussion: 685].

37. Kridel RW, Konior RJ. Irradiated cartilage grafts in the nose. A preliminary report. Arch Otolaryngol Head Neck Surg 1993;119(1):24–30.

38. Burke AJ, Wang TD, Cook TA. Irradiated homograft rib cartilage in facial reconstruction. Arch Facial Plast Surg 2004;6(5):334–41.

39. Adamson PA, Ansari K. Grafts and implants in rhinoplasty – techniques and long term results. Operative Techniques in Otolaryngology-Head and Neck Surgery 2008;19(1):42–58 Friedman C, editor. Elsevier.

40. Schlosser RJ, Park SS. Surgery for the dysfunctional nasal valve. Cadaveric analysis and clinical outcomes. Arch Facial Plast Surg 1999; 1(2):105–10.

41. Sepehr A, Chauhan N, Alexander AJ, et al. Evolution in nasal tip contouring techniques: a 10-year evaluation and analysis. Arch Facial Plast Surg 2011;13(3):217–9.

42. Adamson PA, Zavod M. Changing perceptions of beauty: a surgeon's perspective. In: Chang D, editorvol. 22, 3rd edition. New York: Thieme Medical Publishers Inc; 2006. p. 188–93.

REFERENCES: CONSTANTINIDES

1. Roe JO. The deformity termed 'pug nose' and its correction by a simple operation. NY Medical Record. 1887.

2. Weir RF. On restoring sunken noses without scarring the face. NY Medical Record. 1892.

3. 2011. Available at: http://www.google.com/#hl=en&cp=17&gs_id=1v&xhr=t&q=open+vs+closed+rhinoplasty&pf=p&sclient=psy&source=hp&pbx=1&oq=open+vs+closed+rh&aq=0&aqi=g1g-v3g-ms1&aql=&gs_sm=&gs_upl=&bav=on.2,or.r_gc.r_pw.&fp=29d472dd31b42bb3&biw=1268&bih=693.

4. 2011. Available at: http://www.facialsurgery.com/PPgfaq_nose_open_vs_closed.htm.

5. Toriumi DM, Mueller RA, Grosch T, Bhattacharyya TK, Larrabee WF Jr. Vascular anatomy of the nose and the external rhinoplasty approach. Arch Otolaryngol Head Neck Surg 1996;122(1):24–34.

6. Simons RL. Vertical dome division in rhinoplasty. Otolaryngol Clin North Am 1987;20(4):785–96.

7. Constantinides M, Liu E, Miller PJ, et al. Vertical lobule division in open rhinoplasty: maintaining an intact strip. Arch Facial Plast Surg 2001;3:258–63.

8. Chang CW, Simons RL. Hockey-stick vertical dome division technique for overprojected and broad nasal tips. Arch Facial Plast Surg 2008;10(2):88–92.

9. Godin MS, Waldman SR, Johnson CM. The Use of expanded polytetrafluoroethylene (Gore-Tex) in rhinoplasty: a six-year experience. Arch Otolaryngol Head Neck Surg 1995;121:1131–6.

10. Sykes JM, Patel KG. Use of Medpor implants in rhinoplasty surgery. Oper Techn Otol 2008;19(4): 273–7.

11. Lin G, Lawson W. Complications using grafts and implants in rhinoplasty. Oper Techn Otol 2007;18: 315–23.

12. Byrd HS, Meade RA, Gonyon DL Jr. Use of the autospreader flap in primary rhinoplasty. Plast Reconstr Surg 2007;119:1897–902.

13. Zoumalan R, Shah A, Constantinides M. Quantitative comparison between microperforating osteotomies and continuous lateral osteotomies in rhinoplasty. Arch Facial Plast Surg 2010;12(2):92–6.

14. Constantinides M, Liu E, Miller PJ, et al. Vertical lobule division in open rhinoplasty: maintaining an intact strip. Arch Facial Plast Surg 2001;3: 258–63.

15. Bennet GH, Lessow A, Song P, et al. The long-term effects of alar base reduction. Arch Facial Plast Surg 2005;7(2):94–7.

16. Lee J, Constantinides M. Comparison of long term effects of diced cartilage wrapped with temporalis fascia, Alloderm and Surgicel in rhinoplasty, 1st prize resident presentation (Dr Lee). May 6, 2011 Rhinoplasty Society Meeting. Boston, publication pending.

17. Wise J, Paul B, Alexander A, Constantinides M. Tip projection with maximal medial crural recruitment, in press.

18. Gubisch W. Twenty-five years experience with extracorporeal septoplasty. Facial Plast Surg 2006;22(4): 230–9.

19. Boenisch M, Nolst Trenité GJ. Reconstruction of the nasal septum using polydioxanone plate. Arch Facial Plast Surg 2010;12(1):4–10.

REFERENCES: PEARLMAN

1. Johnson CM, Toriumi DM. Open structure rhinoplasty. W B Saunders Co; 1990.

2. Rethi A. Raccourcissement du nez trop longue. Rev Chir Plast 1934;2:85.

3. Padovan J. External approach to rhinoplasty. Ann Otol Rhinol Laryngol 1966;3:354.

4. Goodman WS. External approach to rhinoplasty. Can J Otolaryngol 1973;2(3):207.

5. Greenough H. Form and function: remarks on art. In: Small HA, editor. Univ of California Press; 1947. In Wikipedia.

6. Sheen JH. Spreader graft: a method of reconstructing the roof of the middle nasal vault following rhinoplasty. Plast Reconstr Surg 1984; 73(2):230.

7. Toriumi DM. New concepts in nasal tip contouring. Arch Facial Plast Surg 2006;8:156.

8. Gruber RP. Malposition of the lower lateral crus: recognition and treatment. Perspect Plast Surg 2001;15(1):33.

9. Constantian MB. Towards refinement in rhinoplasty. Plast Reconstr Surg 1984;74(1):19.

10. Yu K, Kim AJ, Pearlman SJ. Functional and aesthetic concerns of patients seeking revision rhinoplasty. Arch Facial Plast Surg 2010;12(5):291–7.

11. Constantian MB. What motivates secondary rhinoplasty? A study of 150 consecutive patients. Plast Reconstr Surg 2012;130(3):667.

12. Gruber RP, Nahai F, Bogdan MA, et al. Changing the convexity and concavity of nasal cartilage grafts with horizontal mattress sutures: part 1. Experimental results. Plast Reconstr Surg 2005; 115(2):589.

13. Boenisch M, Nolst Trenité GJ. Reconstruction of the nasal septum using polydioxanone plate. Arch Facial Plast Surg 2010;12(1):4–10.

14. Gubisch W. Extracorporeal septoplasty for the markedly deviated septum. Arch Facial Plast Surg 2005; 7(4):218.

15. Kerl R, Stankiewicz J, Weber R, et al. Surgical experience and complications during endonasal sinus surgery. Laryngoscope 1999;109(4):546.

16. Dayan S, Kanodia R. Has the pendulum swung too far? Trends in the teaching of endonasal rhinoplasty. Arch Facial Plast Surg 2009;11(6):414.

17. Simons RL. Vertical dome division in rhinoplasty. Otolaryngol Clin North Am 1987;20(4):785.

18. Adamson PA, Litner JA, Dahiya R. The M-Arch model, a new concept of nasal tip dynamics. Arch Facial Plast Surg 2006;8(1):16.

19. Daniel RK, Calvert JW. Diced cartilage grafts n rhinoplasty surgery. Plast Reconstr Surg 2004;113(7): 2156.

20. Winkler AA, Soler ZM, Leong PL, et al. Complications associated with alloplastic implants in rhinoplasty. Arch Facial Plast Surg 2012; 14(6):437.

21. Cohen JC, Pearlman SJ. Radix grafts in cosmetic rhinoplasty; lessons learned from an 8 year review. Arch Facial Plast Surg 2012;14(6):429.

22. Welling DB, Maves MD, Schuller DE, et al. Irradiated homologous cartilage grafts: long term results. Arch Otolaryngol Head Neck Surg 1988;114(3):291.

23. Kridel RW, Ashoori F, Liu ES, et al. Long-term use and follow-up of irradiated homologous costal cartilage grafts in the nose. Arch Facial Plast Surg 2009; 11(6):378.

24. Guyuron B. Nasal osteotomy and airway changes. Plast Reconstr Surg 1998;102(3):856.

25. Grymer LF. Reduction rhinoplasty and nasal patency change in the cross-sectional area of the nose evaluated by acoustic rhinometry. Laryngoscope 1995; 105(4):429.

26. Helal MZ, El-Tarabishi M, Sabry SM, et al. Effects of rhinoplasty on the internal nasal valve. Ann Plast Surg 2010;64(5):649.

27. McKinney P, Johnson P, Walloch J. Anatomy of the nasal hump. Plast Reconstr Surg 1971;48:528.

28. Rollin RK. Rhinoplasty, an atlas of surgical techniques. New York: Springer; 2004. p. 24.

29. Yoo DB, Jen A. Endonasal placement of spreader grafts: experience in 41 consecutive patients. Arch Facial Plast Surg 2012;14(5):318.

30. Apaydin F. Lateral crural turn-in flap in functional rhinoplasty. Arch Facial Plast Surg 2012;14(2):798.

31. Boahene KD, Hilger PA. Alar rim grafting in rhinoplasty: indications, technique and outcomes. Arch Facial Plast Surg 2009;11(5):285.

Revision Rhinoplasty
Panel Discussion, Controversies, and Techniques

Peter A. Adamson, MD[a,b,*], Jeremy Warner, MD[c,d,*],
Daniel Becker, MD[e,f,*], Thomas J. Romo III, MD[g,*],
Dean M. Toriumi, MD[h,*]

KEYWORDS

- Revision rhinoplasty • Cosmetic surgery • Surgery techniques • Surgical approaches • Rhinoplasty
- Facial rejuvenation • Alloplast • Rib cartilage • Graft • Spreader graft • Graft warp
- Surgical complications

Revision Rhinoplasty Panel Discussion

Peter Adamson, Jeremy Warner, Daniel Becker, Thomas Romo, and Dean Toriumi address questions for discussion and debate:

1. What is the single most difficult challenge in revision rhinoplasty and how do you address it?

2. During revision rhinoplasty, when dorsal augmentation is necessary and septal and ear cartilage is not available, what is the best substance for correcting the problem?

3. If rib cartilage is used for dorsal augmentation during revision rhinoplasty, what is the technique to prevent warping of the graft?

4. Alloplast in the nose – when, where, and for what purpose?

5. Does the release and reduction of the upper lateral cartilages from the nasal dorsal septum always require spreader graft placement to prevent mid-one-third nasal pinching in reductive rhinoplasty?

6. Analysis: Over the past 5 years, how has your technique evolved or what have you observed and learned in performing revision rhinoplasty?

What is the single most difficult challenge in revision rhinoplasty, and how do you address it?

ADAMSON AND WARNER

The single most difficult challenge in revision rhinoplasty is the psychology of the revision rhinoplasty patient. With respect to the psychology of the revision rhinoplasty patient, there is no

---

[a] Adamson Cosmetic Facial Surgery Inc., M110 - 150 Bloor Street West, Toronto, Ontario M5S 2X9, Canada; [b] Department of Otolaryngology - Head and Neck Surgery, University Health Network, University of Toronto, Toronto, Ontario, Canada; [c] Assistant Clinical Professor, Division of Facial Plastic Surgery, University of Chicago, Chicago, IL, USA; [d] NorthShore University Health System, Director of Facial Plastic Surgery, 501 Skokie Boulevard, Northbrook, IL 60602, USA; [e] Becker Nose and Sinus Center, Sewell Medical Center Drive, Suite B, Sewell, NJ 08080, USA; [f] University of Pennsylvania, Philadelphia, PA, USA; [g] The Manhattan Eye, Ear and Throat Hospital, Lenox Hill Hospital, 135 East 74th Street, New York, NY 10021, USA; [h] Division of Facial Plastic and Reconstructive Surgery, Department of Otolaryngology-Head & Neck Surgery, University of Illinois at Chicago, Chicago, IL, USA
* Corresponding authors.
E-mail addresses: paa@dradamson.com (Adamson); jpwmd1@gmail.com (Warner); BeckerMailbox@aol.com (Becker); docromo@romoplasticsurgery.com (Romo); dtoriumi@uic.edu (Toriumi)

Facial Plast Surg Clin N Am 22 (2014) 57–96
http://dx.doi.org/10.1016/j.fsc.2013.09.002
1064-7406/14/$ – see front matter © 2014 Elsevier Inc. All rights reserved.

doubt that the consultative process and partnership with the patient in a revision setting is vastly different from that of the primary rhinoplasty patient. While primary rhinoplasty patients are often hopeful and optimistic, the revision rhinoplasty patient is often hesitant, upset, and leery regarding what can be achieved after a failed attempt to achieve their goals. While it is important to carefully listen to patients' concerns in any consultation, it is especially important to understand the revision rhinoplasty patient's original concerns in addition to their current concerns. In cases where the original concerns can truly no longer be addressed adequately, it is important to be honest with the patient and tell them so. An attempt to lead the patient down a pathway likely to fail is a recipe for disaster for both the patient and the surgeon. We often would like to think we can "save the day," but we must realize what our limits are, especially in the patient who has had 3 or more surgeries. Fortunately, in many cases, the original concerns can be addressed surgically, and it is incumbent upon the surgeon to listen to these concerns and determine what can, and what cannot, be achieved.

Iatrogenic rhinoplasty deformities can come in a variety of shapes and forms. Patient concerns may be focused on the aesthetics of the nose, function of the nose, or both.[1–3] Any deformity may have an impact on the patient. The challenges for the surgeon are to determine:

1. If the deformity is real or imagined
2. If the surgeon has the ability to correct the deformities
3. If the surgeon has the ability to achieve the patient's original goals
4. Whether or not the patient has realistic expectations coupled with the likelihood of satisfaction after surgery.[4–6]

The latter is the most difficult component of the decision making process because it can be unpredictable. But we can make reasonable assumptions during the consultation process based on the patient's personality and demeanor. The patient who understands that surgical outcomes can be partly based on nature and the healing process, and who gives the previous doctor credit for doing their best, can typically be assumed to move forward in an optimistic manner. Conversely, the patient who is very negative regarding their previous doctor, and expresses this in a revision consultation, should be considered cautiously for surgery, as they may be likely to shift their negative feelings toward the new surgeon should there be a suboptimal revision outcome.

BECKER

The nationally reported revision rate for primary rhinoplasty ranges from 8% to 15%.[1–8] Experienced surgeons consistently achieve a high level of satisfaction among their patients. Still, complications can and do occur despite technically well-performed surgery. All surgeons have complications.

The single most important challenge in revision rhinoplasty is to reduce the occurrence of the most commonly seen complications. On a national and international level, the most common complications that I see relate to the midnasal pyramid and lateral alar sidewalls. These complications can be reduced by recognizing this and taking steps to mitigate the risk. In both situations, the key is to ensure strong structural support. For the lateral alar sidewalls, this relates to preserving appropriate support and adding additional support as needed. In the case of the midnasal pyramid, this relates to preserving support after hump reduction. This is discussed further in the final question.

Revision rhinoplasty is a term that encompasses a wide spectrum of technical problems, from straightforward to complex. For the more complicated revision rhinoplasties, in my practice the single most difficult challenge is the psychological aspect.[9] The revision rhinoplasty patient is someone who sought aesthetic improvement and had the opposite result. They are acutely aware of the risks of surgery, they have a strong desire for repair coupled with fear of further worsening. The challenge is to help the patient understand the realistic expectations for surgery, and to empower them to be happy after a successful surgery.

In an established revision practice, patients seeking consultation include many who have all but lost hope. Commonly, the experienced revision surgeon will find that significant improvement is possible. However, to achieve success, it is important that the patient and surgeon come to a realistic understanding of what can and cannot be accomplished. Verbal communication supplemented by computer imaging helps surgeon and patient arrive at a shared surgical goal.

The revision rhinoplasty patient needs an environment in which they will be able to develop and maintain trust. This environment is best created by dedicating oneself to revision surgery, by placing a strong emphasis on patient education, by taking the time necessary to answer the patient's questions and concerns, and by being honest and plain-spoken. The patient must feel that the surgeon has a passion for the operation, and that the surgeon has dedicated him or herself to the pursuit of excellence in nasal surgery, and specifically revision surgery.

I have addressed this challenge by dedicating my practice to nasal surgery. I have created an atmosphere where the patient understands that they are "in the right place." I take the extra time with these patients that they need.

I include them in the process so that they are empowered.

For the most part, the surgical techniques required for a difficult rhinoplasty are available and accessible to the dedicated, experienced and skillful surgeon. This does not ensure success. The current condition of the patient's nose may be the primary limiting factor, and it is important to educate the patient about this. Unexpected problems can be encountered during surgery as well. Ultimately, if the possibility of satisfactory improvement cannot be offered, and/or if the patient is unwilling to accept the risks that are inherent to their surgery, the patient may not be a suitable surgical candidate.

ROMO

The single most difficult challenge in revision rhinoplasty is lengthening the scarred cephalically rotated, shortened nose with absence of vestibular mucosa under the upper lateral cartilages. These problems are often associated with a myriad of other nasal deformities, including internal valve collapse, external valve collapse, overresected dorsum, tip asymmetries, bossa, columella show or retraction, and alar deformities. Each of these

conditions needs to be diagnosed and treated appropriately.

When patients present for an initial revision rhinoplasty consultation, a considerable amount of time – 45 minutes to 1 hour – is allowed. A thorough history of prior nasal surgery is documented. Prior treatment records are obtained if necessary. A complete physical examination of the internal and external nasal structures is completed. The deformities and

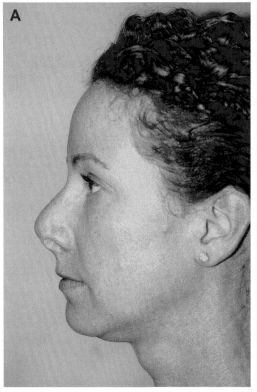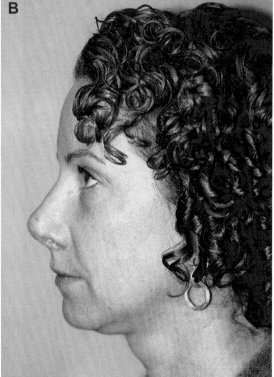

Fig. 1. Romo. Preoperative (*A*) and postoperative (*B*) lateral views of patient who underwent internal reconstruction of vestibular lining and external nasal reconstruction of the overcephalically rotated shortened nose.

problems are then documented on a template. Subsequently, a discussion with the patient commences on the philosophy, complications, benefits and possible treatment plan for the revision rhinoplasty.

Once the extent of the stenosis is determined, the treatment plan proceeds to surgical management. It is well known that lysis of stenosis with stenting using either silastic sheeting or tubing will result in restenosis once the stenting is removed. Therefore relining of the structures is required.

I perform this procedure using a full-thickness skin graft taken from the trichophytic hairline at the mastoid region. An open rhinoplasty technique is employed.[1] The residual upper lateral cartilages are detached from the nasal dorsal septum. Scar tissue lateral to the cartilage is resected. The skin graft is inset at the dorsal septum-nasal bone interface. The skin graft is positioned so the epithelium is facing into the nasal vault. One side of the graft is sutured to the superior nasal septal mucosal line and the alternate edge of the skin graft is sutured to the mucosal lining of the released upper lateral cartilage. This continues inferiorly in a widening manner allowing for expansion of the mid- and lower one-third of the nose. This relining is carried down medially to the septal angle inferiorly and to the superior rim of the planned position of the lower lateral limb cartilage. Structural grafting of the upper lateral cartilages, dorsal augmentation, and lower lateral cartilage reconstruction can then commence. This may entail spreader grafts with caudal extension, caudal septal extension grafts, lower lateral battens, alar rim grafts and columellar augmentation (**Fig. 1**). This structural grafting is doomed to failure unless nasal vestibular lining is replaced, thereby releasing the tethered scarred down nose.

TORIUMI

In my experience the most challenging problem in revision rhinoplasty is correction of soft tissue deformities of the nose. These include cases of skin compromise after necrosis or infection (**Fig. 2**), severe columellar scarring (**Fig. 3**), severe alar notching (**Fig. 4**), and over-resection of the alar

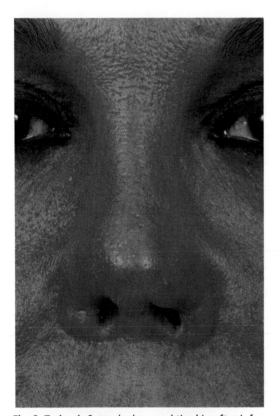

Fig. 2. Toriumi. Severely damaged tip skin after infection and poorly planned vestibular incisions.

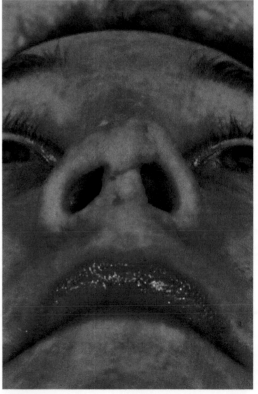

Fig. 3. Toriumi. Revision rhinoplasty challenge. Severe columellar scarring.

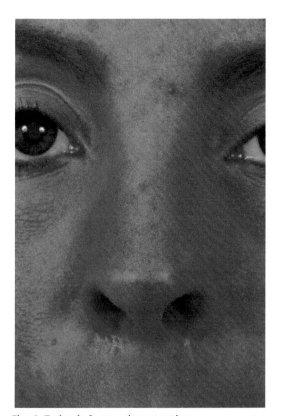

Fig. 4. Toriumi. Severe alar retraction.

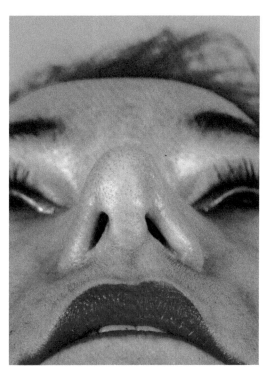

Fig. 5. Toriumi. Revision rhinoplasty challenge. Over-resection of the alar base.

base (Fig. 5). Some of these deformities are associated with the use of alloplastic implants. In such cases of soft tissue deformity it is very difficult to recreate normalcy to the nose. When addressing soft tissue deformities, damaged soft tissues may need to be replaced. Reconstruction is complicated when these soft tissue deformities are in three-dimensionally complex areas of the nose such as the soft tissue triangle or facets (Fig. 6A, B). These areas are very difficult to reconstruction and unfortunately are damaged or deformed from previous surgery more often than I would like to see. To correct these deformities I typically place composite skin cartilage grafts into the site of scar contracture to replace missing vestibular mucosa. This requires creative use of composite grafts taking special care to design grafts to fit the defect and also placement to maximize camouflage of the grafts (see Fig. 6C–G). Despite placement of structural grafts and composite grafts complete correction is rarely possible. These deformities do not fall into the category of typical deformities seen in revision rhinoplasty such as the pinched nasal tip, inverted-V deformity, saddle nose deformity, polly-beak deformity, alar retraction, over-rotated nasal tip,

short nose, hanging columella, and supra-alar pinching. With a normal skin envelope most of these more typical secondary deformities are readily correctable using structural grafting. However, with severe soft tissue defects it is very difficult to completely correct the deformities.

Prevention of soft tissue deformities requires careful positioning of incisions, avoiding closure of the columellar and marginal incision under tension, precise closure of all external and intranasal incisions and conservative alar base reduction. There is rarely a need to make a "rim" incision which is made along the alar margin and introduces a high likelihood for alar notching (Fig. 7). Some surgeons confuse this incision with a marginal incision which is made along the caudal margin of the lateral crura. When performing a delivery approach or external approach one should use a "marginal" incision along the caudal margin of the lateral crura which is at least 3 mm to 5 mm away from the alar rim and moving further away as you move laterally. Surgeons should also avoid making transcolumellar incisions to high on the columella as this can lead to deformity of the soft tissue facets. Ideally the transcolumellar incision should be made at the level of midcolumella or just below midcolumella (Fig. 8).

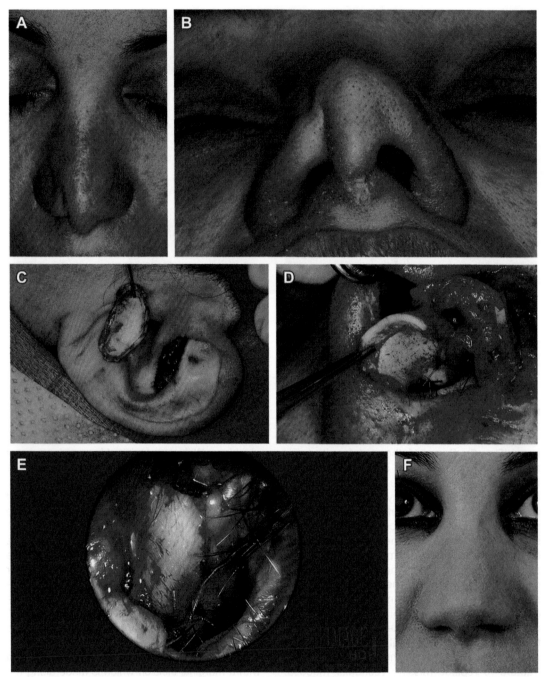

Fig. 6. Toriumi. Patient with severe right alar deformity after infection. (*A*) Frontal view reveals damage to the skin envelope with dimpling and deformity of the soft tissue facet. (*B*) Base view shows the severe contracture in the right soft tissue facet. (*C*) Auricular composite graft of cartilage and overlying skin harvested from the cymba concha. This defect is closed with a full thickness skin graft harvested from the postauricular crease. (*D*) Composite graft is sutured into the defect in the vestibular skin to provide internal lining and allow release of the tissue of the soft tissue facet region. (*E*) Endoscopic view of the composite graft sutured into position. (*F*) Postoperative frontal view showing much improved tip shape and correction of the deformity of the right soft tissue facet region.

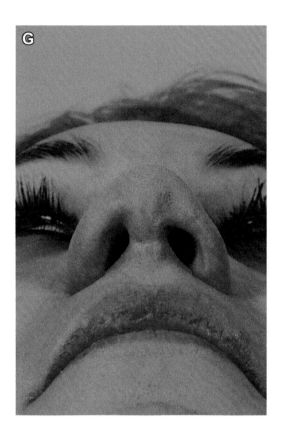

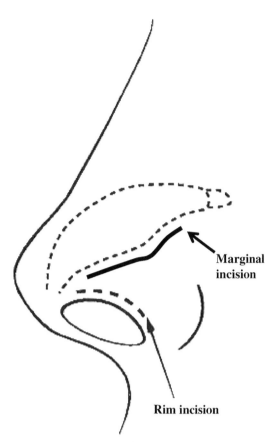

Fig. 6. Toriumi. *(continued) (G).* Postoperative base view showing improved nostril symmetry and correction of the contracture of the right soft tissue facet. Despite the improvement significant asymmetries still are noted. Complete correction of these severe soft tissue deformities is very difficult.

Fig. 7. Toriumi. Marginal incision is made along the caudal margin of the lateral crura. The rim incision is placed along the nostril rim and is fraught with great potential for creating a notched alar margin and should not be confused with the marginal incision.

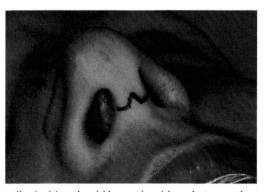

Fig. 8. Toriumi. The transcolumellar incision should be made midway between the top of the nostril and the base of the nose of lower. If the incision is made too high it can create deformity of the soft tissue facet region.

During revision rhinoplasty, when dorsal augmentation is necessary and septal and ear cartilage are not available, what is the best substance for correcting this problem?

ADAMSON AND WARNER

When ear or septal cartilages are not available for rhinoplasty in revision cases, I prefer to use autologous rib cartilage to reshape the nose and maintain its structure (**Figs. 9–12**). Autologous rib cartilage graft harvest is easy, quick, safe, and abundant.[7,8] I can now harvest rib cartilage through a 2 to 3 cm incision in the inframammary crease and it typically only adds about 15 to 20 minutes to the case, making it an equally good donor site compared with other cartilage harvesting options. The perichondrium can also be used as an overlay soft graft to soften any harsh contours. Of course, septal cartilage is an ideal donor

site given the fact that it can be completely hidden and blends into the recovery from the nasal surgery. There is no doubt that rib cartilage grafting does add additional donor site healing pain and scarring. However, pain can be minimized by taking only a portion of the rib,[9] and the scar tends to heal well and is quite well hidden. Some patients presenting for revision rhinoplasty may find the thought of using rib cartilage a foreign and anxiety-provoking concept during my initial consultation with them. After discussing the harvesting process, recovery, and benefits of using this powerful grafting material, patients are uniformly

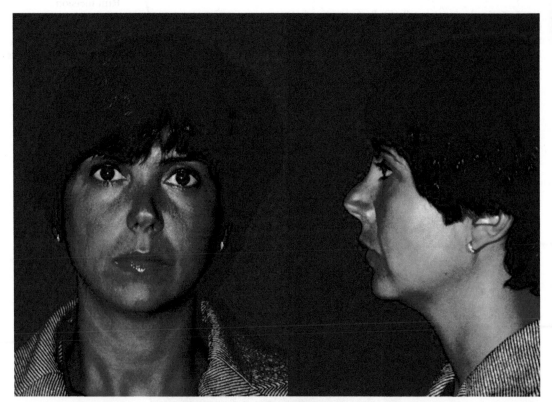

Fig. 9. Adamson and Warner. A 39-year-old female with a significant iatrogenic nasal deformity. She had previously undergone rhinoplasty surgery and had significant dorsal nasal collapse and over-resection. She also had significant polly-beak deformity and tip asymmetry.

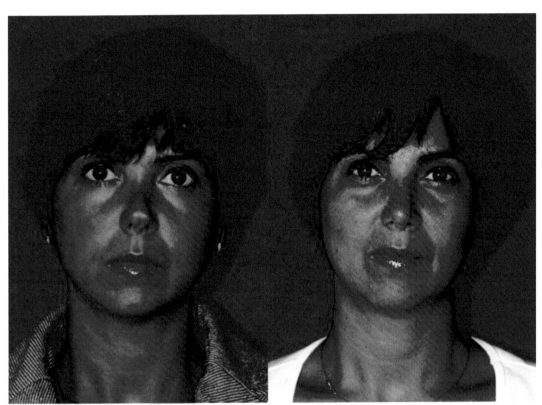

Fig. 10. Adamson and Warner. Pre- and 1 year postoperative anteroposterior (AP) views of patient in **Fig. 1**, before and after autologous rib cartilage grafting to the nasal dorsum and tip.

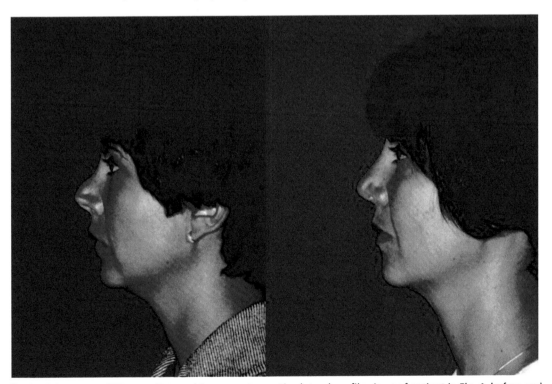

Fig. 11. Adamson and Warner. Pre- and 1 year postoperative lateral profile views of patient in **Fig. 1**, before and after autologous rib cartilage grafting to the nasal dorsum and tip.

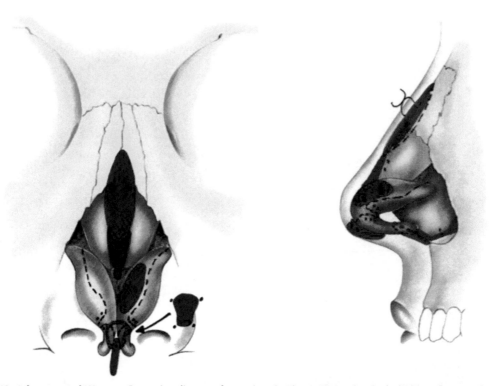

Fig. 12. Adamson and Warner. Operative diagram for patient in **Fig. 1.** Correction included autologous rib cartilage grafting. In addition to tip grafting, an autologous cartilage onlay graft was fashioned, placed in a precise pocket along the nasal dorsum, and secured in place with suture fixation to the underlying cartilaginous skeleton and temporary transcutaneous fixation. The *dashed lines* indicate previously-resected lower lateral cartilage. The *arrow* indicates the actual size and shape of the double infratip cartilage lobule graft secured with perimeter sutures. (*Courtesy of* P.A. Adamson, MD, Toronto, Canada.)

comfortable with the idea and have no problem with this as part of the operative plan.

One of the biggest issues in using rib cartilage is creating the ideal shape. A boat shaped graft, tapering both cephalically and caudally is ideal. I also believe that, in addition to warping being a cause of postoperative aesthetic disappointment, malplacement rather than postoperative displacement is a significant issue. I prefer autologous rib graft over synthetic materials, as I have seen a suboptimal number of patients with synthetic graft-related complications, including infections and extrusions – complications that I have not seen with autologous grafting.[10,11]

BECKER

There is not a single best substance. The literature describes calvarial bone, autogenous rib, autogenous bone-cartilage rib graft, and irradiated rib as options. Alloplasts are also an option. Each option offers risks and benefits. These must be conveyed to the patient, and the surgeon and patient can together make the best choice.

For example, in an older patient with other health issues, in need of significant dorsal augmentation, the additional surgical time and recovery may make an autogenous graft less desirable. In these patients, another issue is that the cartilage of the rib may be calcified and less than ideal. An irradiated rib graft may be the best choice in this situation. Donor site morbidity, reabsorption risk, infection risk, warping, and other risks are all factors that must be weighed and considered with the patient.

On May 4th, 2011 this subject was elegantly discussed and highlighted at the American Academy of Facial and Reconstructive Surgery (AAFPRS)

Advances in Rhinoplasty Course in Chicago, Illinois. In a panel entitled, "My Op Note," distinguished surgeons described 5 different preferred methods for augmenting the dorsum. Each surgeon indicated a preference for their choice of material.

Dr Rollin Daniel described augmentation of the dorsum with diced cartilage. His assistant dices the cartilage so that it can fit through a tuberculin syringe. He creates a tube of deep temporal fascia and injects the diced cartilage into this tube. He then molds it with his sterilely gloved finger and guides it into place with a percutaneous suture. He reported 350 cases in 9 years and stated that he had not seen any resorption of cartilage in these cases.

Dr Dean Toriumi described augmentation of the dorsum with autogenous rib cartilage. He reported that critical points to minimize warping including careful carving, anticipating the bending and carving accordingly, creating a tight pocket for insertion, and fixation to the bony dorsum. He suture secured rib perichondrium to the undersurface of the rib graft, and feels that this is a critical step. At times, a percutaneous K-wire is necessary to facilitate fixation. He reports that there is a significant learning curve to successful autogenous rib grafting.

Dr Peter Hilger described the use of autogenous rib cartilage and bone, harvested from the 11th rib. He similarly feels that stability with bony fusion is key. He favors this graft because it "replaces like with like" and because the risk of warping or bending is mitigated, as bone generally does not warp. He also reports the need for a K-wire at times.

Dr Eduardo Yap reported an extensive experience with alloplasts, specifically with Gore-Tex. He reported over 1000 cases from 2006 to 2009 with only 4 infections, 1 in a primary case and 3 in revisions. He reports that minimizing operating time, and avoiding medial osteotomies/exposure of the intranasal space to the dissection plane, may be a factor in minimizing infection.

Dr Russ Kridel described his extensive use of irradiated rib. He reported long-term follow-up with no difference in absorption compared to autologous rib. He stated that the preparation of the rib was important, that the Tissue Bank must not chemically treat the rib graft.

To summarize, there is no single best choice. Each option offers risks and benefits. These risks and benefits must be conveyed to the patient, and the surgeon and patient can together make the best choice.

ROMO

The plan for dorsal augmentation during revision rhinoplasty is determined during the preoperative evaluation.[2] The loss of dorsal height and width may involve only the middle third of the nose, dorsal bridge cartilage and upper lateral cartilages or may also involve the upper one-third of the nose; ie, nasal bones. Rarely are the nasal bones solely overresected.

If nasal dorsal augmentation is necessary, then autologous tissue is the best grafting material (**Table 1**).[3] The nasal septum is the ideal graft because of its characteristics of providing long-term architectural support. Even if a portion of the septal cartilage is curved, these sections can be incised and carved so that the graft will lay down flat. The obvious drawback is that adequate septal cartilage may not be available because of prior resection.

The next alternative would be auricular cartilage. This includes the concha cymba and concha cavum cartilage. Because of the intrinsic curve in these cartilages, they are difficult to use solely as dorsal onlay grafts. Even if the spring is broken in these cartilages, by cross-hatching and morsalization, they tend to be deficient in length. However, they can be utilized for internal valve spreader grafts.

Without a doubt, during revision rhinoplasty, if dorsal augmentation is required, the ideal grafting material is autologous costo-chondral cartilage. This can be harvested with minimal complications once the technique is mastered. The major difficulty is the actual carving of the graft into its desired shape and having the graft maintain that shape without warping. This problem is so common, that one of the masters of the technique, Dr Jack Gunter, dealt with it by placing a K-wire down the length of the graft in order to prevent warping.[4] Over time, the wire became exposed and had to be removed along with the subsequent warped graft. One of our own contributing authors, Dr Dean Toriumi, designed a technique that lessens this warping process, which will be reviewed during his portion of this discussion.

Table 1
Nonsynthetic grafts

Type	Pros	Cons	Recommended Uses	Comments
Autogenous grafts				
Cartilage				
Septum	Well proven Low extrusion rates Low infection rates Use for structural support and soft tissue augmentation	Limited availability in revision cases	Dorsal onlay, tip grafts, columellar strut, alar batten, soft tissue filler	Gold-standard grafting material
Auricular	Pros similar to septum Concha cymba similar shape to lower lateral cartilage	Limited supply Separate donor site harvest Associated warping	Alar battens, dorsal onlay, tip grafts	—
Costal	Ample supply Similar to septum	Warping Donor site morbidity	Dorsal onlay, tip, columellar grafts, batten grafts, soft tissue filler	Cannot harvest in elderly owing to ossification
Bone				
Split calvarium	Ample supply	Donor site morbidity Resorption Potential of fracture Palpability	Dorsal onlay, columellar strut, alar batten	Not recommended in children
Temporalis fascia	Ample supply	Separate donor site	Soft tissue filler Camouflage grafts	—
Homologous grafts				
Irradiated rib	Ample supply Biocompatibility	Resorption Patient stigma Warping	Dorsal onlay, tip grafts, collumellar strut, alar batten, soft tissue filler	—
Alloderm	Ample supply Biocompatibility	Resorption	Soft tissue filler Camouflage grafts	—

Data from Romo T, Kwak ES. Nasal grafts and implants in revision rhinoplasty. Facial Plast Surg Clin North Am 2006;14:373–87.

TORIUMI

I prefer to use autologous costal cartilage as it is abundant, relatively easy to access, very strong, and predictable to use with good long-term outcomes. By minimizing dissection costal cartilage can be harvested with low morbidity and less pain than with ear cartilage harvest. I prefer to use the sixth rib as it usually lies just under the inframammary crease allowing the incision to be hidden under the breast. Additionally, the sixth rib is surrounded by the fifth and seventh ribs allowing its removal without destabilizing the chest wall and causing pain (**Fig. 13**). The sixth rib is favorable in that one can harvest a relatively long and straight segment for dorsal augmentation. Some patients have a significant genu in the sixth rib which may necessitate using the seventh rib if a long straight segment is needed. I harvest rib cartilage via a 1 cm incision in the right chest (**Fig. 14**).[1–3] Typically the 1 cm incision gets stretched to 1.3 cm (**Fig. 15**). In most cases the incisions heal to the point where they are relatively inconspicuous (**Fig. 16**). I have a very low complication rate, patients have minimal pain, with no instances of pneumothorax.

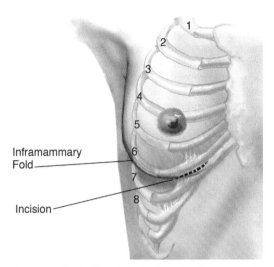

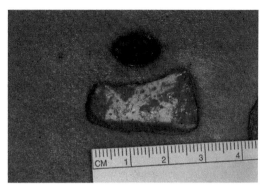

Fig. 15. Toriumi. The chest incision typically stretches to 1.3 cm. A sizeable segment of the sixth rib can be harvested through this incision.

Fig. 13. Toriumi. The sixth rib typically lies under the inframammary crease. An incision can be made in the crease below the breast to hide the incision. The sixth rib can be harvested without destabilizing the chest wall because the 5th and 7th ribs will support the area of dissection.

I prefer not to use any alloplastic implants in the nose as they always have the potential to extrude or become infected.[3] It is true that most implants do fine over the lifetime of the patient. However, when infection or extrusion occurs it can be devastating to the patient frequently creating soft tissue deformities. I also choose not to use irradiated homograft costal cartilage as it does not become vascularized and therefore acts as a non-viable implant. In older patients the costal cartilage can become calcified however it is rare that I am unable to find usable cartilage in most patients. I have also found that rib cartilage in patients who are age 40 to 55 years is less likely to bend or warp. This older cartilage has a brown tint and may be more brittle but is definitely less likely to warp. If a patient has a calcified chest wall I will

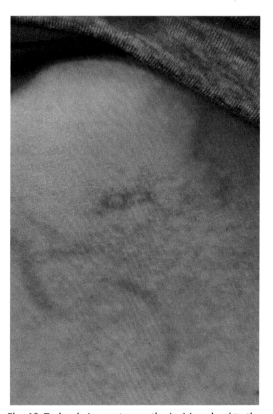

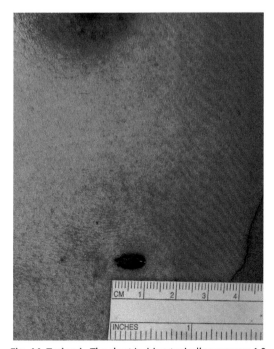

Fig. 14. Toriumi. The chest incision typically measures 1.0 to 1.1 centimeters and lies in the inframammary crease.

Fig. 16. Toriumi. In most cases the incisions heal to the point where they are relatively inconspicuous.

go to the ear for cartilage. In most patients that do not have adequate septal cartilage I will go directly to the chest to harvest costal cartilage as I feel it is a better option for dorsal augmentation.

I have not used the technique of wrapping diced cartilage in fascia for dorsal augmentation.[4] I prefer to use a solid segment of costal cartilage that is precisely carved to create symmetric and well defined dorsal aesthetic lines (brow-tip aesthetic lines). The diced cartilage in fascia does not have the same structural integrity as a solid piece of rib cartilage and therefore is not able to create the same definition to the dorsal lines. I also believe that the diced cartilage can deform or change shape over time potentially leading to an unfavorable contour. We do not have enough data on the long-term efficacy of this technique and if there is any resorption over time. Additionally, there is chance that thinner skin will contract leading to a "cobble stoning" effect.

Using costal cartilage for dorsal augmentation is associated with a significant learning curve. Harvesting the costal cartilage is not complicated. It is the planning, carving of the graft, placement into a tight midline pocket and rigid fixation that require precise execution. Using this technique one can create a natural appearing nasal dorsum that also feels natural as they are not moveable.

If rib cartilage is used for dorsal augmentation during revision rhinoplasty, what is the technique to prevent warping of the graft?

ADAMSON AND WARNER

Many techniques have been used to prevent cartilage graft warping.[12] I have found that warping of autologous rib cartilage varies greatly among different patients. I have found it frustrating in the past to think that I'm allowing the cartilage to soak en-bloc for a long period of time, only to find that it warps within minutes of cutting it into grafts. I no longer find it sufficient to simply excise the perichondrium and allow the block to soak. I will, therefore, anticipate what grafts I will need to the extent possible, harvest the cartilage, excise the perichondrium, cut the cartilage into grafts, and then soak them in saline for 30 minutes while I perform the open rhinoplasty approach and prepare the nose for cartilage graft placement. I will also tend to use slightly thicker grafts in my current practice, as I find that I tend to get less warping doing so. Once the grafts have been cut, significant warping can be a challenge, as the cartilage tends to be more resistant to scoring at this point. Horizontal mattress sutures can be used to straighten the cartilage as well. Fortunately, there tends to be ample donor site material, and should a graft warp beyond its use during soaking, a second graft can often be fashioned from the remaining cartilage. Should I run into a situation where all of the graft material has warped beyond use, it can be diced up and wrapped in fascia and used for augmentation grafting.[13–15]

I have tended to use a percutaneous suture cephalically and transfixion sutures caudally through the caudal aspect of the middle third of the nose and the cartilage to fix the grafts in place. I have also done some rasping of the bone to help with fixation. In my experience, it seems more difficult in younger patients to prevent warping. Some individuals have tried to use a combination of bone and cartilage, with the bone being placed cephalically, to minimize this. I have not done this.

BECKER

The technique of balanced cross-sectional carving is the cornerstone. This has been well described. A careful, patient carving technique may be the best approach. The fact that the placement of K-wires has been advocated as a consideration to reduce warping speaks to the fact that, even in experienced hands, the risk of warping cannot be prevented or eliminated, but only mitigated.

At the Advances in Rhinoplasty course in Chicago, Illinois on May 5, 2011, Toriumi reported that in his hands, critical points to minimize warping including careful carving, anticipating the bending and carving accordingly, creating a tight pocket for insertion, and fixation to the bony dorsum. He suture secures rib perichondrium to the undersurface of the rib graft, and feels that this is a critical step. At times, a percutaneous K-wire is necessary to facilitate fixation.

ROMO

One of the intrinsic problems with utilizing rib carti-lage is the tendency of this graft to warp. There-fore, the surgical management to prevent this process is to break the tensile forces of the carti-lage. This is accomplished first by harvesting a portion of a costal rib (number 7, 8 or 9), which has a straighter intrinsic pattern. Next, the rib graft is placed in a warm saline bath, which causes the graft to bend in directions that are unique to each graft. Once these patterns are noted, the graft is carved longitudinally. A long central core graft is produced. This process eliminates the perichon-drium, which can pull the graft toward this lining. The graft is then again placed in a warm saline

bath, left for several minutes, and then retrieved. If additional warping is noted, the graft can be incised transverse to the length, ie, hot dog cuts break the intrinsic bends.

If all this fails to produce a straight rib graft, then a K-wire can be placed down the length of the graft.[4] This wire is placed just short of the distal edge of the rib graft, and the proximal wire is clip-ped at the alternate rib graft end. Ultimately, even with all these maneuvers being performed, the rib graft may have some warping in the long-term healed nose. It is just one of the sequelae that you bring to the table in using rib graft for dorsal augmentation.

TORIUMI

Warping is always a concern when using costal cartilage. This can be particularly problematic when using costal cartilage for dorsal grafts. The reason for the propensity for warping of dorsal grafts is that the costal cartilage dorsal graft is typically placed onto the dorsum of the nose and is not fixated and is free to bend or move.[1,2] When rib grafts are placed deep in the tissues (spreader grafts, struts, etc.) they are less likely to warp or bend as there are forces counteracting the tendency to bend or deform.[3]

We minimize problems with dorsal grafts by identifying the tendency for the graft to bend and implant the graft so the concave side of the graft is placed against the nasal dorsum (**Fig. 17**).[1–3] We do not use straight grafts for the dorsum as it

is imperative to identify the tendency to bend and by placing the concave side of the graft into a tight subperiosteal pocket the tendency to bend is counteracted by the fixation and overlying skin envelope.[1–3]

The other key to avoiding bending or warping is to fixate the dorsal graft as rigidly as possible to the nasal dorsum.[1–3] This is accomplished by making a very tight subperiosteal pocket over the nasal dorsum. Then perichondrium harvested from the surface of the harvested rib is sutured onto the undersurface of the dorsal graft (**Fig. 18**). Prior to positioning the dorsal graft a 2 mm straight osteotome is used to make many perforations in the dorsal nasal bones to create sites of exposed cortical bone that will promote fixation to the perichondrium sutured to the dor-sal graft. An alternative is to rasp the bone mak-ing sure the rasp does not increase the width of the dorsal pocket. After making the perforations in the bone or rasping, the dorsal graft with peri-chondrium is pushed into the tight dorsal pocket (**Fig. 19**).[1–3] Strips of perichondrium can also be placed along the sides of the dorsal graft to mini-mize the chances of visualizing the edges of the dorsal graft. A minimum of 2 5-0 PDS sutures are used to fixate the dorsal graft to the upper lateral cartilages of the middle nasal vault as well. We have found the dorsal graft will rapidly fixate to the nasal bones limiting movement of the dorsal graft. With fixation of the dorsal graft to the nasal dorsum movement or bending is much less likely.

In some cases a tight pocket is not possible over the nasal dorsum. In these cases a transcutaneous 0.45 threaded Kirschner wire can be used to fixate

Fig. 17. Toriumi. The dorsal graft is curved to make sure the tendency to bend is identified. With this bend identified the concave side of the graft is placed down against the nasal dorsum into a tight pocket so the force of the skin envelope acts against the grafts tendency to bend.

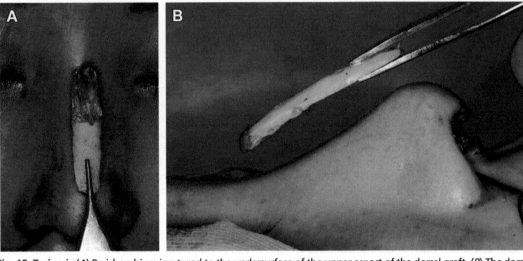

Fig. 18. Toriumi. (*A*) Perichondrium is sutured to the undersurface of the upper aspect of the dorsal graft. (*B*) The dorsal graft is then placed into a tight subperiosteal pocket and placed directly against the perforated bone of the nasal dorsum. This will force the dorsal graft with perichondrium against the perforated bone to aid in fixation of the graft.

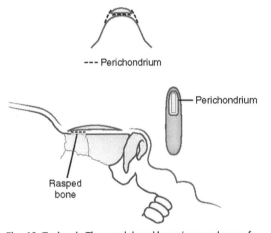

Fig. 19. Toriumi. The nasal dorsal bone is rasped or perforated with a 2 mm straight osteotome to create a rough surface to fix to the perichondrium that is sutured to the undersurface of the dorsal graft. This promotes rigid fixation of the dorsal graft to the underlying nasal dorsum and decrease the chance of movement or warping.

the dorsal graft with perichondrium to the underlying perforated bone (**Fig. 20**).[3] Another option is to drill a hole across the nasal bones and pass a suture that passes over the dorsal graft and is cinched down to fixate the graft to the nasal bones.[3]

I believe the key to avoiding warping or bending of costal cartilage dorsal grafts is to promote fixation to the bony dorsum.[1–3] If the dorsal graft is immobilized any tendency to bend will be minimized. Patients also feel the rigidly fixed dorsal graft will look and feel more natural (**Fig. 21**).

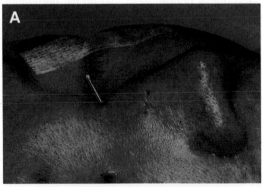
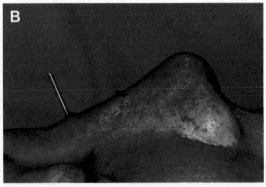

Fig. 20. Toriumi. Patient that had Silastic implant removed has a large dorsal pocket necessitating fixation of the dorsal graft with perichondrium to the bone using a threaded K-wire that is placed through a small stab incision over the nasal dorsum and through the dorsal graft and into the underlying bone. The K-wire can be removed in the office on the 7 postoperative day.

A

B

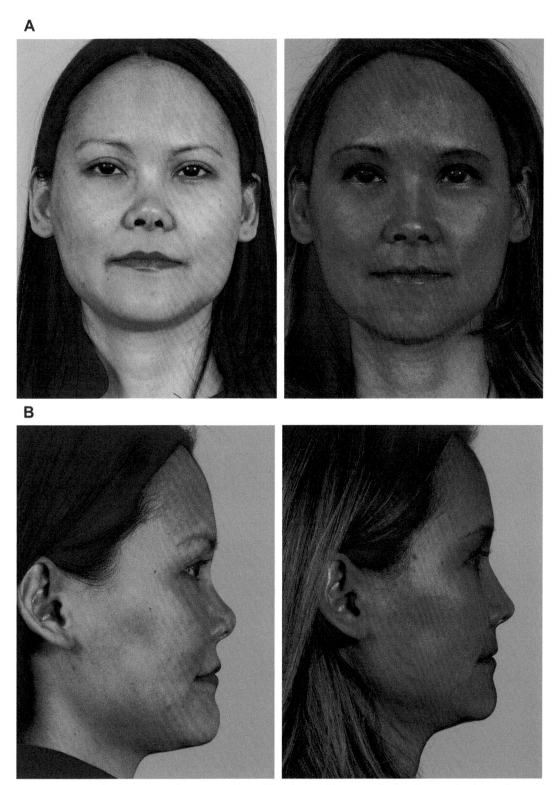

Fig. 21. Toriumi. This patient underwent revision rhinoplasty with removal of a GoreTex implant. The nasal dorsum was then reconstructed using a costal cartilage dorsal graft with attached perichondrium. (*A*) Preoperative and postoperative frontal views showing improved brow tip aesthetic lines and less nostril show. (*B*) Preoperative and postoperative lateral views showing raised nasal dorsum and counter-rotation of the nasal tip.

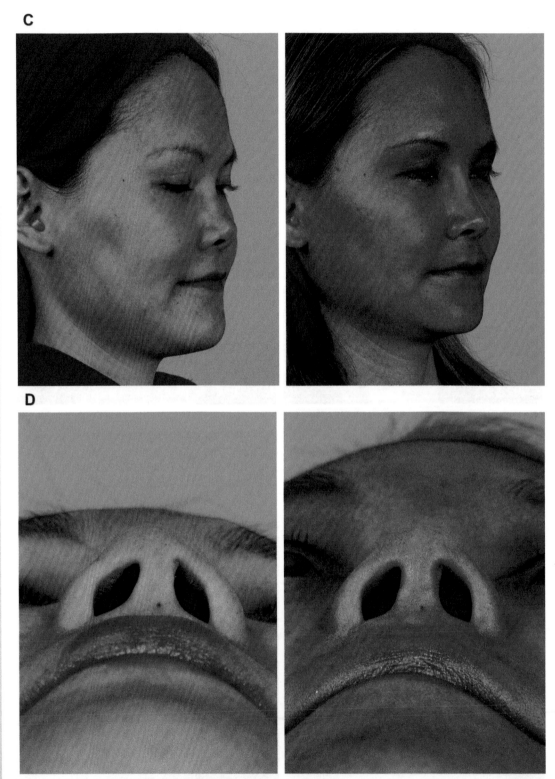

Fig. 21. Toriumi. (*continued*) (*C*) Preoperative and postoperative oblique views showing improved dorsal line. (*D*) Preoperative and postoperative base views showing improved nasal tip symmetry.

Does the release and reduction of the upper lateral cartilages from the nasal dorsal septum always require spreader graft placement to prevent mid-one-third nasal pinching in reductive rhinoplasty?

ADAMSON AND WARNER

The short answer to this is "No." I do not typically find a need to place spreader grafts in cases where the dorsum has not been significantly reduced. If the reduction is minimal, the junction of the upper lateral cartilages beneath the nasal bones at the rhinion may leave a smooth rounded rhinion. In my practice, I almost always release the upper lateral cartilages from the nasal dorsal septum, in order to expose the septum for correction and cartilage harvesting, and also to allow true reduction of the dorsal septum for dorsal contouring. There are many patients who require reduction of the upper lateral cartilages as part of the operative plan, in order to reduce fullness in the middle third, from either the anterior-posterior view, from the profile view, or from both. Whether or not spreader grafting will be required prior to securing the upper lateral cartilages back to the septum simply depends on the internal anatomy at the time of repair, and also on the aesthetic appearance from the external view, which requires thoroughly expressing the edema to the extent possible and double-checking your work.[16,17]

If there is a need to reduce the upper lateral cartilages, it is important to point out that this should not be done until the osteotomies are completed, as the upper lateral cartilages will drop down a bit after the nasal bones are repositioned. If the upper lateral cartilage is reduced prior to the osteotomies, one may find that the cartilages are now too short after the bone has dropped down into its new position. Also, the upper lateral cartilages can be reduced either vertically (which will narrow the middle third a little bit) or horizontally (which will lower their vertical height more), or a combination of both. In particular I try to minimize the amount of vertical reduction near the rhinion as this may cause more pinching of the upper lateral cartilages as they heal. Often after significant dorsal reduction and/or upper lateral cartilage reduction, a spacer graft is indicated at the rhinion. I would define a spacer graft as one that simply fills the space of the open roof, as opposed to a spreader graft, which really works to actually lateralize the upper lateral cartilage from the septum. A spreader graft is therefore used to either widen the nose aesthetically or support upper lateral cartilages, which are collapsing, and open the internal valve. Additionally, spreader grafts may be used unilaterally or bilaterally and may be longer or

shorter. If being placed cephalically, they tend to more fill the open roof or prevent cephalic inflare of the upper lateral cartilages, whereas caudally they are used again aesthetically or to improve the internal valve. Spreader grafts can be placed a millimeter or 2 below the dorsal profile of the dorsal septal strut in order to avoid apparent widening of the nose.

With respect to the internal anatomy at the time of repair, once the upper lateral cartilages are reduced and the dorsum has been appropriately contoured, one must look to see whether or not securing the upper lateral cartilages to the septum is going to cause excessive pinching and reduction. This can sometimes be seen throughout the middle third and it is especially important to assess this in the internal valve region. It is important to carefully inspect the rhinion directly when doing the open approach, as the swelling of the skin-soft tissue envelope may well hide the anatomic open roof, collapse of the upper lateral cartilages or pinching caused by cephalically placed transfixion sutures in the middle third.

Also on internal exam, one must make sure that the 2 sides are symmetric, especially if they were symmetric to begin with. In most rhinoplasties where the nose is fairly straight to begin with, the angle of divergence of the upper lateral cartilages to the septum will also need to be as symmetric as possible. Of course, this may not be true for the crooked nose. I am quite thorough in evaluating the functional nasal status pre-operatively, including the internal nasal valve function. And I have found that patients with any suggestion of internal nasal valve incompetence may require spreader grafting if I feel the upper lateral cartilages are too pinched during the procedure.

From a purely aesthetic standpoint, I have found that while creating an ideal internal anatomy is often important, it is the final external appearance that must be ensured prior to final closure. I will do this by manually squeezing the nasal dorsum and sidewalls with a wet sponge to ensure that the edema is removed and the actual contour can be seen. This will give the surgeon the best "final appearance" of the nose and any adjustments can be made accordingly. If the nose does appear to be pinched in the middle third, it must be determined whether or not a spreader/spacer graft or an onlay graft must be placed. If pinching is seen, the internal anatomy should be examined. Any apparent narrowing of the middle third at this point can be treated with a spreader/spacer graft. If the middle third internal anatomy appears adequate and there is still external apparent pinching, then an onlay graft would be more appropriate. I prefer to use a transcutaneous suture to secure middle third onlay grafts, and have found excellent reliable results doing this, in addition to being a much easier operative maneuver than securing the graft to the underlying skeleton.

BECKER

No, the release and reduction of the upper lateral cartilages from the nasal dorsal septum does NOT always require spreader graft placement. Countless thousands of patients have had endonasal rhinoplasty with hump reduction without nasal valve collapse. At the AAFPRS Advances in Rhinoplasty Course on May 4, 2011, Pastorek described his technique of careful, calibrated reduction of the dorsum via an endonasal approach with meticulous preservation of the underlying mucosa, which he reports act as "mucosal spreader grafts." He reported that with over 30 years of surgical practice, he has not encountered pinching of the middle nasal vault as a significant problem with his approach. This has been the experience of many other experienced endonasal surgeons.

The important philosophical concept is the emphasis on anatomic diagnosis and preservation of supportive structures. Still, middle third nasal pinching after hump reduction remains a risk. The experience of Perkins is telling.

Perkins[10] describes an evolution in his personal philosophy that reflects some of the issues

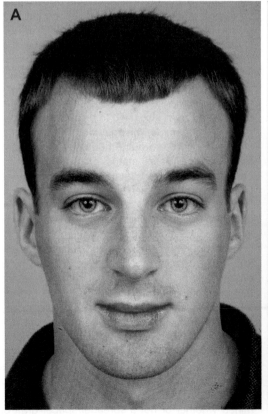 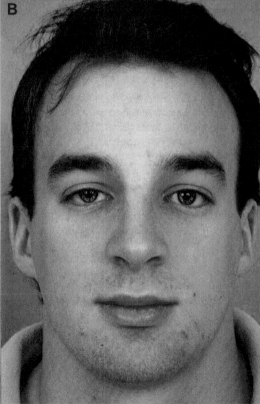

Fig. 22. Becker. Hump reduction can be achieved via an endonasal approach. Pre and 1 year postoperative photos.

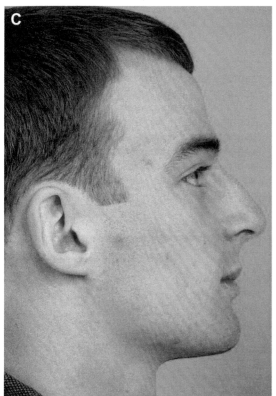

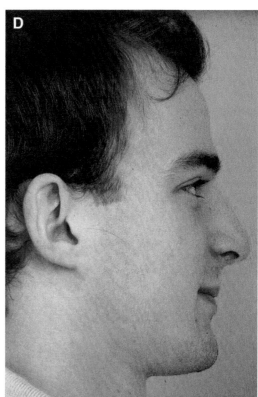

Fig. 22. Becker. (*continued*)

involved in the decision making process, and provides valuable insight into the evolution in the decision making that has occurred over the last 15 to 20 years. While the concept of a graduated approach to achieve a pleasing aesthetic result has been foremost in his personal philosophy, the evolving need to achieve more refined results and prevent late complications has resulted in his increased use of spreader grafts after hump reduction, which he does via the open approach, which he feels facilitates this grafting. Perkins continues to strongly advocate the philosophy that the approach selected should provide the least intervention in the shortest time to achieve a satisfactory result and satisfy the patient's goals. However, his choice of approach has changed due to late complications that he has seen occur. The 2 areas that he found most commonly cause late complications in rhinoplasty are the midnasal pyramid and lateral alar sidewalls. Paramount to preventing the late complications in the middle vault is to provide a structural foundation for the middle vault (ie spreader grafts). While issues such as these can be addressed using the endonasal approach, it is sometimes far easier to place structural grafts via the external approach (**Figs. 22 and 23**).

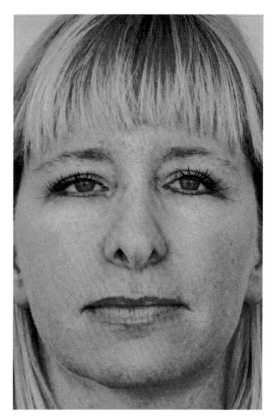

Fig. 23. Becker. There is a risk of an inverted-V deformity, such as the one seen here, when a hump reduction is performed and the upper lateral cartilages do not have adequate support. As a practical matter, it is easier to place spreader grafts to support the upper lateral cartilages via an external approach.

ROMO

I think this question is presenting several scenarios. First, is it necessary to release the upper lateral cartilages (ULCs) from the dorsal septum in order to perform dorsal reduction?

Over the last 25 years, I have seen the reduction rhinoplasty technique continue to evolve. Initially, complete release of the ULCs, with incision and release of the internal nasal mucosa, along with aggressive resection of the ULCs and dorsal septum, was performed. This was the standard procedure in New York for the last 50 years and is still being performed by some surgeons today. The sequelae of this technique led to long-term healing scenarios that produced the classic inverted V at the rhinione. Additionally, a pinched and collapsed lower mid-one-third nasal contour was produced that essentially closed off the internal nasal valve.

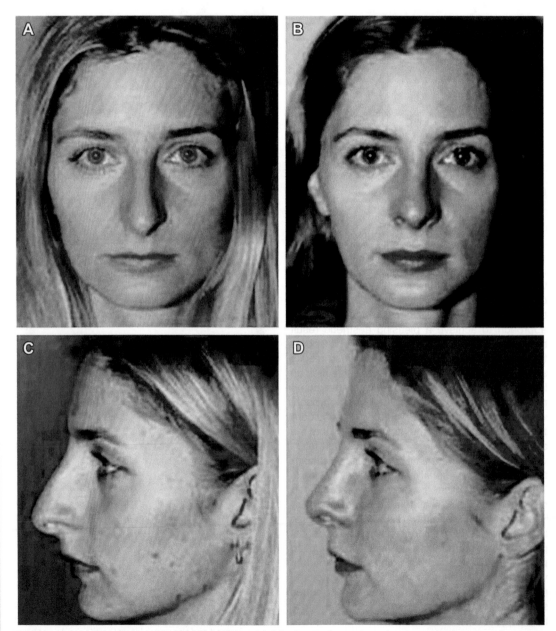

Fig. 24. Romo. Preoperative frontal (*A*) and lateral (*C*) views of a tethered nose requiring spreader grafts. Postoperative frontal (*B*) and lateral (*D*) views of reduction structured rhinoplasty with spreader grafts.

The recognition of these aesthetic and functional nasal problems has led to the present technique. This procedure advocates less dorsal cartilage resection and not violating the underlying internal dorsal mucous membrane. In addition, resuturing of the ULCs to the dorsal septum and the placement of dorsal spanning sutures have become standard.

Either way, both of these techniques require release of the upper lateral cartilages from the dorsal septum. Since the majority of reduction rhinoplasties are performed utilizing one of these techniques, the question then becomes, do all rhinoplasties require spreader grafts to prevent any pinching of the mid-one-third of the nose? Theoretically, I would then say 'Yes.' The reality of the situation is that in the majority of reduction rhinoplasties performed today, spreader grafts are not placed.

Therefore, I believe that this requirement is instituted on a case-by-case basis, predicated upon the preoperative examination of the nose. There are classic preoperative nasal profiles that indicate a higher incidence of having significant postoperative nasal pinching. These patients present with shortened nasal bones and a very high and thin mid-one-third nasal dorsum. This extends from the rhinione to the septal angle. In addition, these noses are usually overprojected and have a long nasal spine; ie, the classic tethered nose. In this case scenario, following proper reduction of the nasal dorsum, spreader grafts should be paced to prevent lower-mid-one-third nasal pinching (**Fig. 24**).

TORIUMI

I prefer to place spreader grafts when the upper lateral cartilages are divided from the dorsal septum. I find that structural reconstruction of the middle nasal vault results in better long-term outcomes with symmetric favorable dorsal aesthetic lines (**Fig. 25**).

I do believe there is a variable need for spreader grafts depending on the anatomy encountered in the patients. Patients that have long nasal bones are less likely to have problems with middle vault collapse as longer nasal bones are associated with shorter upper lateral cartilages (**Fig. 26**).[5] Patients that have long nasal bones do not have sufficient length in the upper lateral cartilages to exhibit collapse. In patients with long nasal bones the importance of spreader grafts is diminished as their effect on upper lateral cartilage position is less significant. On the other hand, patients with short nasal bones will have longer upper lateral cartilages that are much more likely to collapse infero-medially and result in middle vault collapse and an inverted-V deformity.[5]

Skin thickness also plays a role in the preservation of the dorsal aesthetic lines after rhinoplasty. Patients with thin skin are likely to show even small degrees of collapse of the upper lateral cartilages. Patients with thick skin may not show any external signs of middle vault collapse even though they may have functional compromise and inferomedial collapse of the upper lateral cartilages. Therefore, patients with long nasal bones and thick skin are the least likely to need spreader grafts as they will likely not show any aesthetic problems if some collapse occurs.

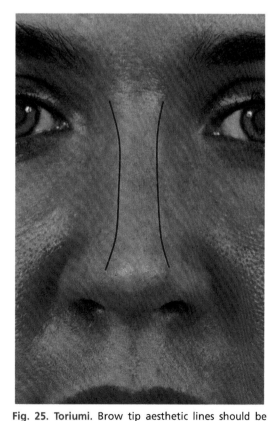

Fig. 25. Toriumi. Brow tip aesthetic lines should be symmetric but curvilinear. Creating symmetrical dorsal aesthetic lines requires reconstruction of the middle nasal vault in most cases where the upper lateral cartilages have been divided from the dorsal septum.

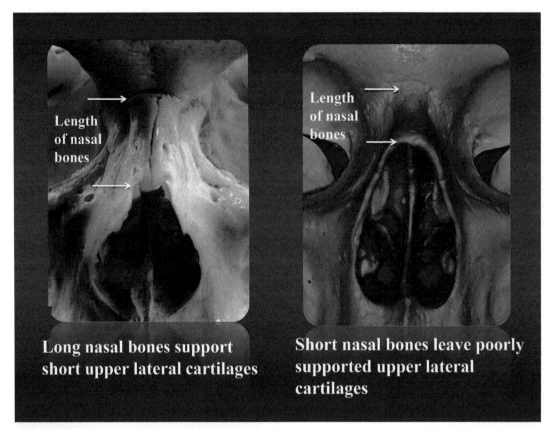

Fig. 26. Toriumi. Patients with long nasal bones are less likely to demonstrate collapse of the middle nasal vault as the upper lateral cartilages are well supported. On the other hand patients with short nasal bones will have longer upper lateral cartilages that may become flail and collapse infero-medially after dorsal hump reduction.

Alloplast in the nose – when, where, and for what purpose?

ADAMSON AND WARNER

The senior author (PAA) has used a number of alloplasts for dorsal augmentation over many years. These have included Supramid mesh, silicone, Mersilene mesh and more lately expanded polytetrafluoroethylene. We have found a 7% incidence of malpositioning, postoperative displacement, or infection or extrusion requiring removal. The alloplasts were often very effective, very smooth and when they worked well, they worked well for long periods of time (**Figs. 27–31**). I, along with many others, also have tried absorbable alloplasts such as vicryl mesh, alloderm and gel foam over the years. It is my impression that in the vast majority of cases there really was never any scar tissue replacement of these materials, and that at the end of the day they provided very little if any value in reconstructive rhinoplasty.

The use of synthetic grafts has been well described,[18–23] and I have certainly seen beautiful

results with synthetic grafts. There is no doubt that these grafts can provide for an optimal aesthetic appearance. However, I would argue that the same can be done with autologous cartilage material without the higher risk of infection and extrusion. While I have seen many beautiful results, I have seen some dramatic complications with these materials, especially in terms of extrusion. I have removed many extruding silicone implants from the nose, which leave permanent and often disfiguring scars, in addition to some significant skin defects. I have ended up treating many of these patients like a Mohs reconstruction patient, and many of them require local flaps to fill in substantial defects where the implants have extruded. Because there is no such thing as an autologous cartilage shortage in any patient, and because septal, ear, and rib cartilage can all be harvested with ease, this has become my preferred method today.

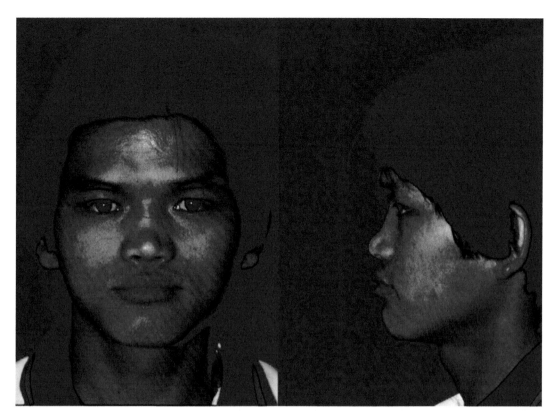

Fig. 27. Adamson and Warner. A 23-year-old male with congenital nasal deformity including deficient dorsal and tip projection, ill-defined dorsal aesthetic lines, and lack of tip definition.

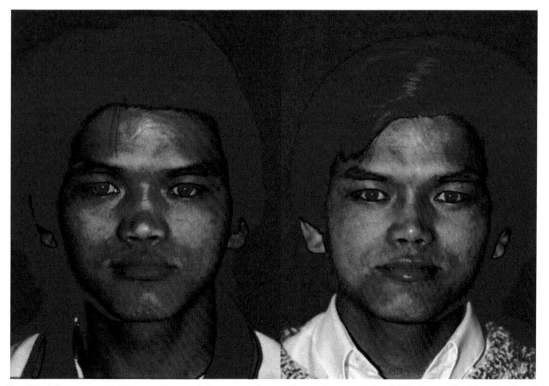

Fig. 28. Adamson and Warner. Pre- and 1 year postoperative anteroposterior (AP) views of patient in **Fig. 4**, before and after silicone augmentation implants to the dorsum, tip, and columella.

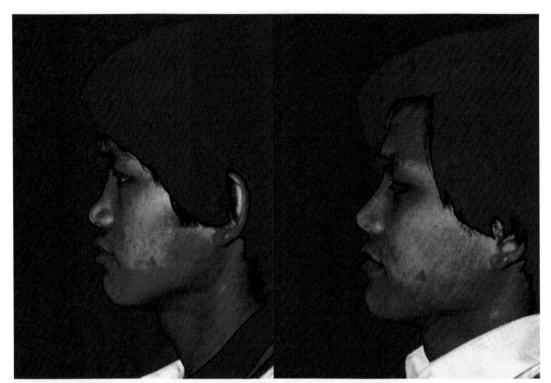

Fig. 29. Adamson and Warner. Pre- and 1 year postoperative lateral views of patient in **Fig. 4,** before and after silicone augmentation implants to the dorsum, tip, and columella.

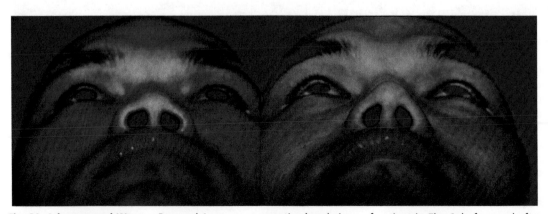

Fig. 30. Adamson and Warner. Pre- and 1 year postoperative basal views of patient in **Fig. 4,** before and after silicone augmentation implants to the dorsum, tip, and columella.

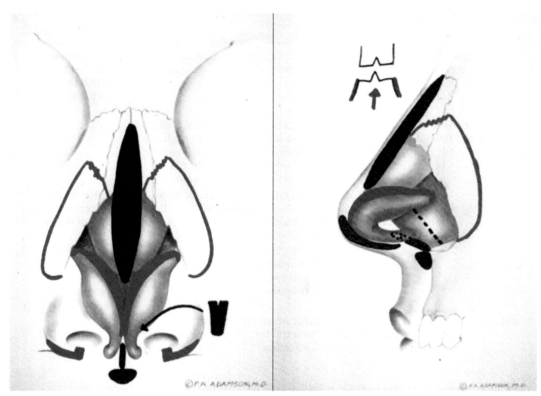

Fig. 31. Adamson and Warner. Operative diagram for patient in **Fig. 4**. Correction included silicone dorsal augmentation implant and silicone columellar and tip augmentation implants. In addition to silicone implant augmentation, other refinements included bilateral cephalic trims, osteotomies, alar base reductions, and columellar advancement flaps to allow tension-free closure after increased projection is attained. The *dashed line* indicates absent caudal septum to this position. The *arrow* indicates the placement of the (actual size) infratip and tip shield-type graft.

BECKER

I have never used an alloplast in rhinoplasty. They clearly have a place in rhinoplasty, as they are widely used throughout the world, and especially in Asian rhinoplasty. I have certainly seen the devastating effect on the skin-soft tissue envelope when an alloplast has become infected and extruded through the skin. I discuss and offer alloplasts as an option with patients when explaining the various alternatives.

ROMO

The utilization of alloplastic implants for nasal augmentation elicits varied responses from educators in the rhinoplastic surgery arena. Many, in fact, advocate a total ban on all alloplastic implants in rhinoplasty. The dictum is predicated upon the documented fact that alloplasts have an increased complication rate compared to autologous grafting material in revision rhinoplasty (**Table 2**).[3] Autologous grafts for revision rhinoplasty include septal cartilage, auricular cartilage and costo conchal cartilage in that sequence.[5] Additionally, irradiated homologous costal cartilage (IHCC) has been utilized over the last 30 years and goes in and out of fashion. Proponents of IHCC emphasize the large quantity of grafting material available and the lack of donor site morbidity as reasons for its use. On the other hand, unpredictable resorption and warping of the graft have been noted in long-term follow-up studies.[6] Additionally, the graft can be significantly expensive. There are no perfect nasal implants. The ideal implant bears the following features (**Box 1**).[3]

Be that as it may, alloplastic implants in the modern era, have been used for nasal augmentation rhinoplasty for at least 40 years.[7] Solid silicone silastic implants were the first modern implant utilized. This implant can be used as a dorsal component, or dorsal tip component with or without a columella strut.[8]

Table 2
Synthetic implants

Type	Pros	Cons	Recommended Uses	Comments
Expanded-porous polytetrafluoroethylene (Gore-Tex)	Allows tissue ingrowth Biocompatible Soft/pliable Sculptable	Poor structural support	Dorsal onlay, tip grafts	Not recommended in patients with a septal perforation
Porous high-density polyethylene (Medpor)	Allows tissue ingrowth Biocompatible Sculptable	Difficult to remove Palpability Challenge to insert	Dorsal onlay, tip grafts, columellar strut, alar batten	—
Silicone Solid form (Silastic)	Easy to insert Soft/pliable Sculptable Biocompatible	Extrusion potential Capsule formation No tissue ingrowth Lifetime risk of extrusion	Dorsal onlay	Reliable results limited to use in thick skin (Asians)
Injectable form (Adatosil-5000, Silikon-1000)	Permanence	Potential for local and systemic response	Subtle soft tissue defects	Not US Food and Drug Administration approved for use as soft tissue filler
Mersilene	Soft/pliable Low resorption Allows tissue ingrowth	Difficult to remove Potential for infection	Soft tissue augmentation Dorsal onlay, tip graft, premaxilla graft	—
Temporary soft tissue fillers (Restylene, Radiesse)	Ease of use	Temporary	Subtle soft tissue defects	—

Data from Romo T, Kwak ES. Nasal grafts and implants in revision rhinoplasty. Facial Plast Surg Clin North Am 2006;14:373–87.

Box 1
Features of the ideal nasal reconstruction material

- Inert
- Easy to sculpt
- Mimics color and consistency of tissue it replaces
- Resistant to trauma
- Resistant to infection
- Resistant to extrusion
- Mechanically stable with respect to surrounding tissues
- Readily available
- Inexpensive
- Easy to remove
- Sterilizable
- Can be used for structural support and to replace lost soft tissue volume

Data from Romo T, Kwak ES. Nasal grafts and implants in revision rhinoplasty. Facial Plast Surg Clin North Am 2006;14:373–87.

A significant drawback of this material is that a fibrous capsule is always formed around this implant. This process essentially allows the implant to be slightly free-floating in its healed position.[9]

Because the implant is not biointegrated into the local soft tissue, even minimal nasal trauma can result in this implant becoming exposed and necessitate removal.

Even with this characteristic, silastic nasal implants are utilized globally for nasal augmentation because they are relatively inexpensive and easy to obtain.[10]

Expanded polytetrafluoroethylene (ePTFE) (Gore-Tex; W.L. Gore & Associates) implants allow for slight soft tissue infiltration, which helps stabilize the implant from future nasal trauma.[11] Additionally, the soft texture of the implant makes for ease of carving of the implant. Once in place, the soft nature of the implant camouflages well on visualization and on palpation of the nose. On the other hand, this implant cannot be used for strong structural support in areas where this is required.[12] Furthermore, it is very expensive. Porous high-density polyethylene (pHDPE) (Medpor; Porex Technologies) implants allow for aggressive ingrowth of soft tissue into the implant. This implant is approximately 50% porous, and over time, progressive infiltration and stabilization of the implant is noted.[13]

However, the harder, firmer nature of the pHDPE implant can also be its main drawback. Even with soft tissue infiltration, nasal trauma can lead to implant exposure, infection and the need for implant removal. In areas of poor vascular supply, this material like all implants has a greater incidence of complications and should be utilized with caution.[14]

TORIUMI

I have never used an alloplast in the nose because I feel I always have a better option in some form of autologous cartilage. It is very rare that I am not able to find septal, auricular or costal cartilage for grafting purposes. Obviously there should always be some costal cartilage available unless the chest wall is completely calcified. If I encounter an older patient with a calcified chest wall I would consider using irradiated homograft rib. If there is no septum or ear left I will perform a needle palpation of the patients rib in the office. I inject some local anesthetic over the sixth and seventh ribs and then insert a 1.5 inch 27 gauge needle into the chest down to the rib (**Fig. 32**).[1] I first identify the sixth rib with my fingers then insert the needle down to that rib (see **Fig. 32**A). I can then walk the tip of the needle up and down the rib to assess the degree of calcification (see **Fig. 32**B). I find this maneuver very reliable as one can determine the degree of calcification of the rib and locate the bony junction laterally. I also perform this maneuver intraoperatively before making any incision in the chest to harvest rib to rule out excessive calcification. Special care must be taken when doing this maneuver to avoid passing through the rib or between the ribs as this can result in a pneumothorax.

I do understand that alloplastic implants do well in most patients that are implanted, however, I still prefer autologous cartilage. The nose is mobile and relatively unprotected. I believe autologous materials are usually going to do better in the mobile nose and better handle trauma and aging.

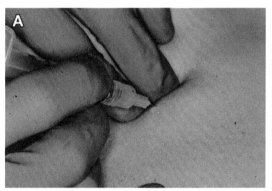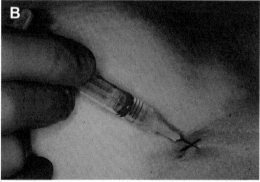

Fig. 32. Toriumi. To assess the degree of calcification of the rib cartilage a 1.5 inch 27 gauge needle can be passed through the skin of the chest and down to the rib cartilage. The needle can be used to penetrate the rib cartilage move along the rib to detect areas of calcification. This can be very helpful to determine if harvestable cartilage is available in the older patient. Additionally, the needle can be used to identify the osseocartilaginous junction. Care must be taken to avoid passing too deep and penetrate the pleura as this can result in a pneumothorax.

Analysis: over the past 5 years, how has your technique evolved or what have you observed and learned in performing revision rhinoplasty?

ADAMSON AND WARNER

The primary concept that has evolved over time with respect to revision rhinoplasty is that of structural re-building. The concept of "less is more" does not typically lend itself to most revision rhinoplasty surgeries. There are certainly some revision cases where a small adjustment is needed in order to take a reasonable result to an exceptional result. The majority of revision rhinoplasties, however, require strong structural re-building and reconstruction in most cases. Scar tissue, poor structural support, significantly deformed anatomic structures, and a less pliable skin envelope create an environment where insufficient structural change will result in a suboptimal revision result, disappointment, and further revision surgery. It is often necessary to have to make the decision to invoke significant structural changes in the native cartilages, and often even necessary to abandon the native cartilages altogether and re-build and reconstruct the optimal structures using cartilage grafting. I have found that making the structures stronger and having the knowledge, experience, and courage to reconstruct portions of the nose that are

unsalvageable in their current state leads to long lasting satisfactory results that will get the patient to the place he or she intended to achieve in the first place.

Having said this, it has been a lifetime lesson to come to learn that up to about the third rhinoplasty procedure, you can frequently alter the actual dynamics of the nasal cartilages with sculpting, suturing and grafting techniques. However, once you are into your fourth or higher number of revisions, in my experience the scar tissue and technical manipulations of the previous procedures make it almost impossible to actually expect any dynamic change. At this point the procedure much more becomes one of simply reduction, augmentation and supporting tissues without any real expectation of dynamic improvement in the function of the nose.

BECKER

I have observed that at times, complications occur in surgery that has been well performed.

Performing revision rhinoplasty has taught me valuable lessons in reducing complications in rhinoplasty. By seeing the unfortunate results that can occur from various surgical interventions, I have translated that into steps to reduce or

mitigate complications. I believe that should be the primary lesson from the study of revision rhinoplasty.

That is to say, since the most common problem I see in the tip relates to over-resection, the lesson to learn is to be more preservative in primary tip rhinoplasty (**Fig. 33**).

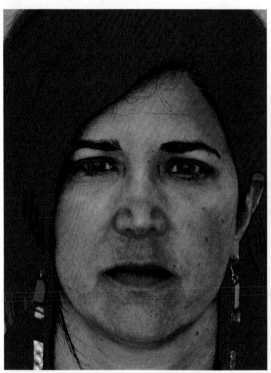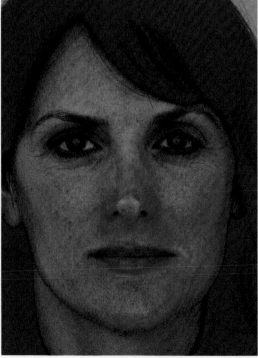

Fig. 33. Becker. Over-resection of the nasal tip cartilages can lead to significant aesthetic and functional deformities.

I see dorsal irregularities and over-resection of the bony nasal bridge as common issues in patients seeking revision rhinoplasty. I have focused some energy on instrumentation used in this area, and I am a strong advocate of powered rasps and disposable osteotomes. In particular, it is important to realize that osteotomes for resection of the bony hump dull with use. Professional sharpening, and also sharpening by the surgeon with a sharpening stone, may not return the edge to its original sharpness. A dull osteotome may be a factor in over-resection of the bony hump, as the deeper bone is thinner than the more superficial bone. A dull osteotome may be a factor in the creation of dorsal irregularities as well. The surgeon may wish to consider replacing their osteotomes, or returning it to the manufacturer for sharpening, after a limited number of uses.

It is important that the revision surgeon approach the nose with an emphasis on risk management. Surgery is not an exact science and the results are not always predictable. The surgical plan is designed to achieve the shared surgical goals with as little trauma as possible. Still, the patient is reminded that complications can still occur, and that not all complications are correctible.

Ultimately, success in revision rhinoplasty is based on well-developed judgment, wisdom, and accumulated knowledge and experience. Like most surgeries, revision rhinoplasty is both a science and an art. Skill comes from experience and wisdom, combined with a measure of talent. The revision surgeon must have a detailed understanding of the multiple anatomic variants encountered. The surgeon must also have accumulated the appropriate surgical techniques and experience. Specifically, the revision surgeon must acquire knowledge of the surgical alterations that occur, and how to achieve an improvement or correction when the result is undesirable. This second skill set is acquired by careful follow-up of operated patients over time.

ROMO

What I have learned over the past many years is that there are still a considerable number of surgeons who continue to perform rhinoplasty incorrectly. They are limited to an almost non-existent understanding of the need to maintain nasal function post-rhinoplasty surgery. This problem is continued when these surgeons solely utilize a reductive rhinoplasty technique, despite the advances and trends in primary and functional rhinoplasty made during the last 2 decades.

Such a myopic approach can produce asymmetric, weakened nasal architecture that may then become distorted as the overlying skin heals down to the nasal structures (**Fig. 34**).

The tensile forces of the skin-healing process contacts little of the underlying weakened

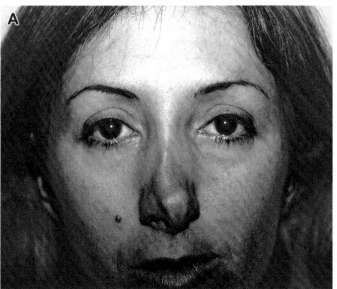
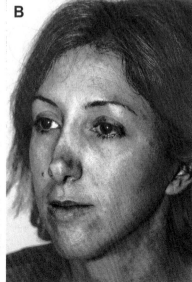

Fig. 34. Romo. Frontal (*A*) and oblique (*B*) views of postoperative deformity of overresected rhinoplasty.

architecture and therefore continues to constrict. This leads to long-term healing scenarios, 3 to 5 years, which were commonly noted in the past. Therefore, aggressive reductive rhinoplasty techniques can lead to aesthetic deformities and a compromise of nasal respiratory function.

A second observation is that following a discussion of revision rhinoplasty with an adult female patient. Once the discussion turns to the subject of the need to augment the nose in order to improve nasal function and cosmetic appearance, the patient's reaction and retort are interesting: "Does this mean that my nose will be bigger? (reply: "Yes") No way!" This has resulted in the patient not proceeding with revision rhinoplasty, or in requesting modifications being performed that

eliminate a process to enlarge the nose even if not doing so produces a lesser global nasal result. Occasionally, the patient will proceed with an alternate facial rejuvenation procedure and eliminate the revision rhinoplasty altogether (**Fig. 35**). I do not view this situation as an untenable position and/or mandate my total treatment plan for the revision rhinoplasty be accepted by the patient. If I can provide improvement in the nose aesthetically by utilizing a partial or limited procedure, I will consider that option when the patient understands there will be a limited improvement in function. I perceive this as a customization of the revision rhinoplasty and will proceed if the patient understands that the ultimate limited result will be our goal.

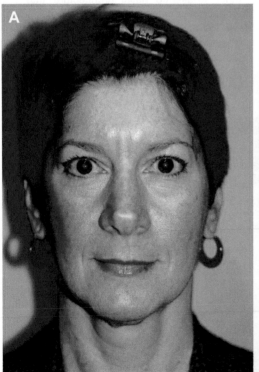
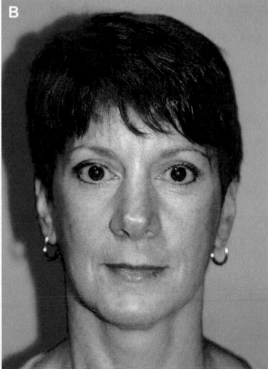

Fig. 35. Romo. Patient with overresected rhinoplasty with additional brow and midface ptosis (preoperative frontal [A] and lateral [C]), corrected by an endoscopic brow and midfacelift (postoperative frontal [B] and lateral [D]).

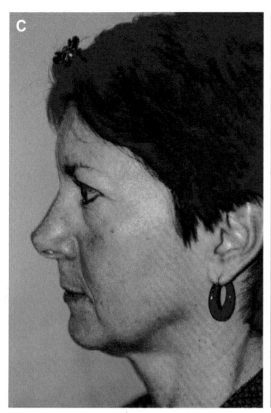 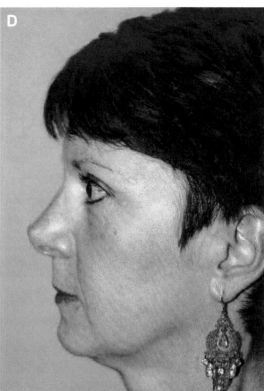

Fig. 35. Romo. (*continued*)

TORIUMI

This is a very complex question as my technique has evolved greatly over the past 5 years. For the purposes of brevity, I will focus on 3 changes in my technique of revision rhinoplasty.

1. I have shifted almost exclusively to using costal cartilage in secondary rhinoplasty patients unless there is an intact septum. If there is an intact septum I will try to use the septal cartilage for the structural grafting. At the time of injection of local anesthetic agent into the nose I will use the needle to palpate the septum and I can usually determine if septal cartilage is present. If there is no septal cartilage I will go directly to the chest to harvest the costal cartilage. I have also gone to the 1 cm incision in the past 5 years as well. I have found this to be very appealing to the patients as they are left with minimal scarring from the rib cartilage harvest. I use a larger 1.5 cm to 2 cm incision in patients that are older and less concerned about the scar and in patients that require harvesting a segment of rib longer than 4 cm or if more than 1 rib is needed. I moved to using thinner

smaller costal cartilage grafts in the nose to keep the nose softer and less stiff. This helps to minimize the stiffness in the nose and upper lip that can be seen in patients that undergo costal cartilage grafting to the nose.

2. I have gone to repositioning the lateral crura with lateral crural strut grafts in a large percentage of patients undergoing secondary rhinoplasty (**Fig. 36**).[6,7] This technique entails dissecting the remnant of the lateral crura free from the underlying vestibular skin and suturing lateral crural strut grafts to the undersurface.[8] The lateral crura are then repositioned into a position that best contours the nasal tip and alar margins. This technique is very powerful for controlling nasal tip contour, position of the alar margin and provides tremendous support to the lateral wall of the nose. I use this technique for increasing and decreasing tip projection to lessen the need for shield tip grafts. I find this technique is very versatile and allows me to control many parameters to tip shape and position.[9] There is a proportionately large percentage of revision patients that

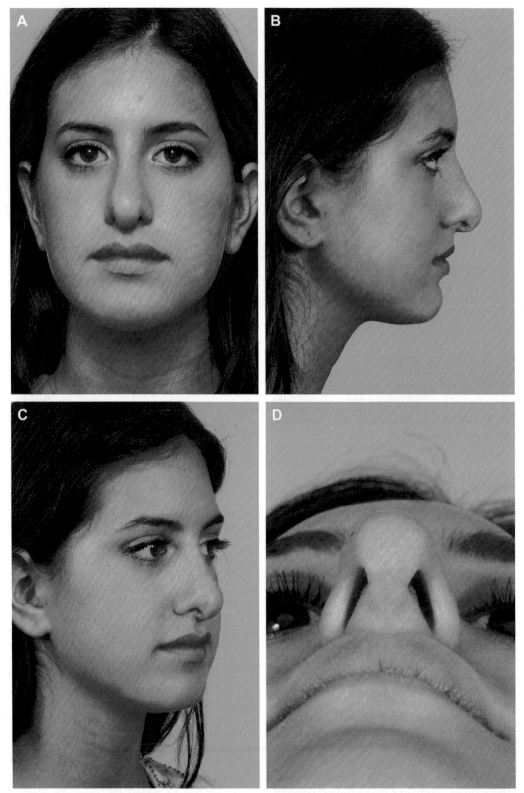

Fig. 36. *Toriumi.* This patient underwent previous rhinoplasty resulting in deformity. She has a prominent hanging columella and bulbous nasal tip. (*A*) Frontal view reveals a prominent tip lobule that is contributing to a dependent tip and a bulbous asymmetric nasal tip. (*B*) Lateral view reveals a hanging tip lobule. (*C*) Oblique view reveals a hanging tip lobule. (*D*) Base view reveals a wide columella and external nasal valve collapse.

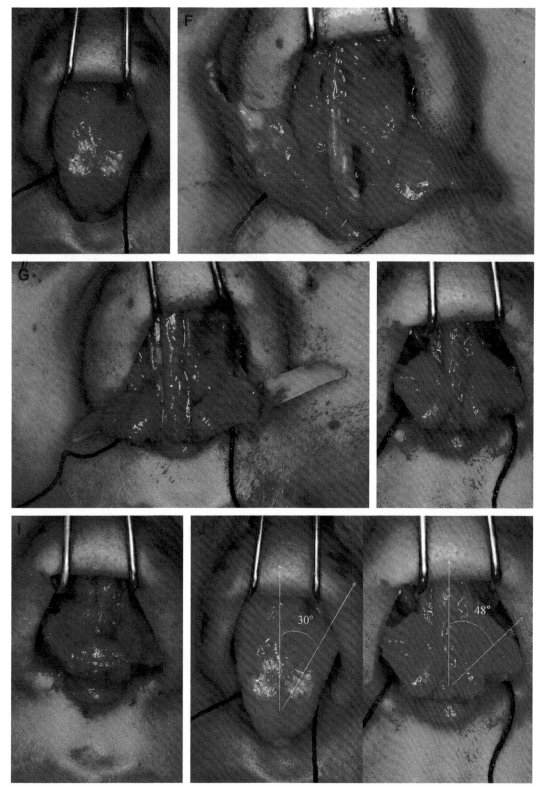

Fig. 36. (*continued*) (*E*) Intraoperative view of the lower lateral cartilages reveals cephalically positioned lateral crura. (*F*) The lateral crura have been dissected from the underlying vestibular skin. (*G*) Septal cartilage lateral crural strut grafts have been suture fixated to the undersurface of the remnant lateral crura. (*H*) The lateral crura remnants with the lateral crural strut grafts have been repositioned and placed into caudally positioned pockets. (*I*) Horizontally oriented onlay tip graft is sutured to the domes. (*J*) Left: Preoperative positioning of the lateral crura showing an angle off of midline of 30 degrees. Right: After repositioning the lateral crura into caudally positioned pockets the angle of the lateral crura off of midline is now 48 degrees which is more favorable.

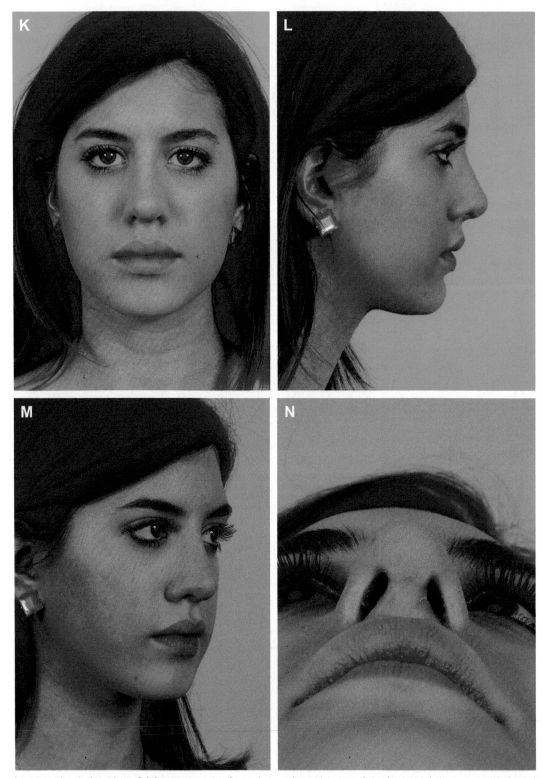

Fig. 36. Toriumi. (*continued*) (*K*) Postoperative frontal view shows improved tip shape and a more appropriate tip lobule. (*L*) Postoperative lateral view shows improved columellar lobule angle and correction of the hanging tip lobule. (*M*). Postoperative oblique view shows an improved tip contour. (*N*) Postoperative base view shows improved symmetry.

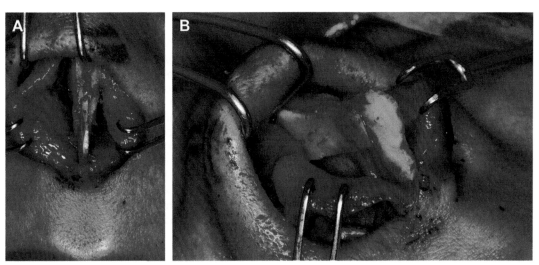

Fig. 37. Toriumi. Caudal septal extension graft. (*A*) Costal cartilage caudal septal extension graft placed end to end and stabilized with extended spreader grafts. (*B*) Note how the caudal septal extension graft is longer anteriorly and shorter inferiorly to control nasal tip rotation.

have cephalically positioned lateral crura (**Fig. 36**E). This deformity can be corrected by dissecting the lateral crura from the underlying vestibular skin (see **Fig. 36**F). Then lateral crural strut grafts are sutured to the undersurface of the lateral crura (see **Fig. 36**G). Pockets are dissected to allow repositioning the lateral crura into a more caudal position (see

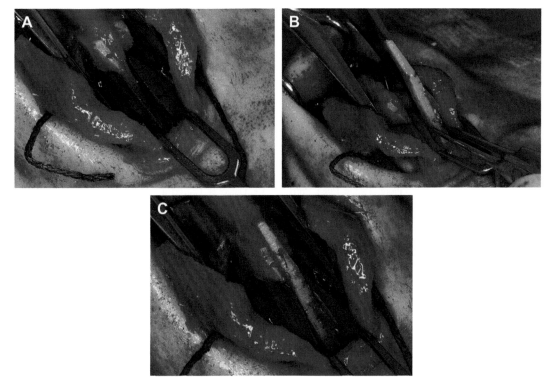

Fig. 38. Toriumi. (*A*) Spreader grafts are not long enough to stabilize the caudal septal extension graft. A 0.25 mm PDS plate is used to stabilize the caudal septal extension graft. Small holes can be made in the PDS plate with a 16 gauge needle to allow vascular ingrowth into the cartilage and also to promote fibrosis to stabilize the graft. (*B*) The caudal septal extension graft is placed end to end. (*C*) Once in position the caudal septal extension graft provides excellent nasal tip support.

Fig. 36H). Then a horizontally oriented onlay tip graft can be sutured over the domes for additional tip definition (see **Fig. 36**I). With repositioning the lateral crura can be moved from an unfavorable angle (less than 30 degrees of midline) to a favorable angle (greater than 35 degrees) (see **Fig. 36**J).[9]

3. I have moved away from columellar struts to almost exclusive use of caudal septal extension grafts placed end to end. In the past I overlapped septal extension grafts but found it to occasionally block the airway.[10] To stabilize the end to end septal extension grafts I use extended spreader grafts that extend beyond the existing caudal septum to fixate the extension grafts (**Fig. 37**).[1,6,7] The caudal septal extension grafts provide excellent nasal tip support and precisely control nasal tip position. When repositioning the lateral crura it is imperative that the nasal tip be strongly supported to avoid torqueing of the nasal tip when the lateral crura are moved. The caudal septal extension grafts provide the necessary support and are an integral part of the reconstruction. If extended spreader grafts are not available and cartilage is scarce I will use a 0.25 mm resorbable PDS plate (Mentor Worldwide) with holes made in the plate to promote vascular ingrowth and fibrosis (**Fig. 38**).[11] The PDS plates resorb over 6 months leaving the septal extension graft in good position. In some instances I will fix the septal extension graft to the nasal spine to provide maximal support. However, rigid fixation of the extension graft to the nasal spine can create a stiff upper lip and can alter the patient's smile. Patients may note a crease in the upper lip when they smile if the extension graft is fixed to the nasal spine. Therefore, fixation to the nasal spine is limited to severe cases of the ptotic nasal tip, severe deficiency in caudal septal support and congenital cleft lip rhinoplasty patients with premaxillary deficiency.

There are many other modifications that I have made in my technique for secondary rhinoplasty. The 3 changes noted above are the most significant and have improved my outcomes.

REFERENCES: ADAMSON AND WARNER

1. Sinno H, Izadpanah A, Thibaudeau S, et al. The impact of living with a functional and aesthetic nasal deformity after primary rhinoplasty: a utility outcomes score assessment. Ann Plast Surg 2012;69(4):431–4.
2. Yu K, Kim A, Pearlman S. Functional and aesthetic concerns of patients seeking revision rhinoplasty. Arch Facial Plast Surg 2010;12(5):291–7.
3. Thomson C, Mendelsohn M. Reducing the incidence of revision rhinoplasty. J Otolaryngol 2007;36(2):130–4.
4. Davis R, Bublik M. Psychological considerations in the revision rhinoplasty patient. Facial Plast Surg 2012;28(4):374–9.
5. Adamson P, Litner J. Psychologic aspects of revision rhinoplasty. Facial Plast Surg Clin North Am 2006; 14(4):269–77.
6. Chauhan N, Alexander A, Sepehr A, et al. Patient complaints with primary versus revision rhinoplasty: an analysis and practice implications. Aesthet Surg J 2011;31(7):775–80.
7. Moon B, Lee H, Jang Y. Outcomes following rhinoplasty using autologous costal cartilage. Arch Facial Plast Surg 2012;14(3):175–80.
8. Moshaver A, Gantous A. The use of autogenous costal cartilage graft in septorhinoplasty. Otolaryngol Head Neck Surg 2007;137(6):862–7.
9. Chauhan N, Sepehr A, Gantous A. Costal cartilage autograft harvest: inferior strip preservation technique. Plast Reconstr Surg 2010;125(5):214e–5e.
10. Park J, Jin H. Use of autologous costal cartilage in Asian rhinoplasty. Plast Reconstr Surg 2012;130(6): 1338–48.
11. Won T, Jin H. Immediate reconstruction with autologous cartilage after removal of infected alloplast in revision rhinoplasty. Otolaryngol Head Neck Surg 2012;147(6):1054–9.
12. Kim D, Shah A, Toriumi D. Concentric and eccentric carved costal cartilage: a comparison of warping. Arch Facial Plast Surg 2006;8(1):42–6.
13. Daniel R, Calvert J. Diced cartilage grafts in revision rhinoplasty. Plast Reconstr Surg 2004;113(7):2156–71.
14. Tabbal N, Tepper O. Diced cartilage versus solid grafts in rhinoplasty. Aesthetic Plast Surg 2011;35(4):580–1.
15. Unlu R, Altun S, Inozu E, et al. Diced cartilage grafts in rhinoplasty surgery: current techniques and applications. Plast Reconstr Surg 2009;124(2):666.
16. Pearlman S, Baratelli R. Avoiding complications of the middle vault in rhinoplasty. Facial Plast Surg 2012;28(3):310–7.
17. Sykes J. Management of the middle nasal third in revision rhinoplasty. Facial Plast Surg 2008;24(3):339–47.
18. Stelter K, Strieth S, Berghaus A. Porous polyethylene implants in revision rhinoplasty: chances and risks. Rhinology 2007;45(4):325–31.
19. Inanli S, Sari M, Baylancicek S. The use of expanded polytetrafluoroethylene (Gore-Tex) in rhinoplasty. Aesthetic Plast Surg 2007;31(4):345–8.

20. Romo T, Kwak E. Nasal grafts and implants in revision rhinoplasty. Facial Plast Surg Clin North Am 2006;14(4):373–87.

21. Baran C, Tiftikcioglu Y, Baran N. The use of alloplastic materials in secondary rhinoplasties: 32 years of clinical experience. Plast Reconstr Surg 2005;116(5):1502–16.

22. Romo T, Sclafani A, Jacono A. Nasal reconstruction using porous polyethylene implants. Facial Plast Surg 2000;16(1):55–61.

23. Godin M, Waldman S, Johnson C. Nasal augmentation using Gore-Tex. A 10-year experience. Arch Facial Plast Surg 1999;1(2):118–21.

REFERENCES: BECKER

1. Kamer FM, Pieper PG. Revision rhinoplasty. In: Bailey B, editor. Head and neck surgery otolaryngology. Philadelphia: Lippincott; 1998. p. 2291–302.

2. Rees TD. Postoperative considerations and complications. In: Rees TD, editor. Aesthetic plastic surgery. Philadelphia: Saunders; 1980.

3. McKinney P, Cook JQ. A critical evaluation of 200 rhinoplasties. Ann Plast Surg 1981;7:357.

4. Thomas JR, Tardy ME. Complications of rhinoplasty. Ear Nose Throat J 1986;65:19–34.

5. Tardy ME, Cheng EY, Jernstrom V. Misadventures in nasal tip surgery. Otolaryngol Clin North Am 1987; 20:797–823.

6. Simons RL, Gallo JF. Rhinoplasty complications. Facial Plast Surg Clin North Am 1994;2:521–9.

7. Becker DG. Complications in rhinoplasty. In: Papel I, editor. Facial plastic and reconstructive surgery. 2nd edition. New York: Thieme; 2002. p. 452–60.

8. Tardy ME. Rhinoplasty: the art and the science. Philadelphia: Saunders; 1997.

9. Becker DG. Revision rhinoplasty: personal philosophy. In: Becker DG, Park SS, editors. Revision rhinoplasty. New York: Thieme; 2009. p. 189–201.

10. Perkins SW. The evolution of the combined use of endonasal and external columellar approaches to rhinoplasty. Facial Plast Surg Clin North Am 2004;12:35–42.

REFERENCES: ROMO

1. Gunter JP, Rohrich RJ. External approach for secondary rhinoplasty. Plast Reconstr Surg 1987;80: 161.

2. Acarturk S, Arslan E, Demirkan F, et al. An algorithm for deciding alternative grafting materials used in secondary rhinoplasty. J Plast Reconstr Aesthet Surg 2006;59:409–16.

3. Romo T, Kwak ES. Nasal grafts and implants in revision rhinoplasty. Facial Plast Surg Clin North Am 2006;14:373–87.

4. Gunter JP, Clark CP, Friedman RM. Internal stabilization of autogenous rib cartilage grafts in rhinoplasty: a barrier to cartilage warping. Plast Reconstr Surg 1997;100:161–9.

5. Cardenas-Camarena L, Guerrero MT. Use of cartilaginous autografts in nasal surgery: 8 years of experience. Plast Reconstr Surg 1999;103:1003–14.

6. Clark JM, Cook TA. Immediate reconstruction of extruded alloplastic nasal implants with irradiated homograft costal cartilage. Laryngoscope 2002; 112:968–74.

7. Berghaus A, Stelter K. Alloplastic materials in rhinoplasty. Curr Opin Otolaryngol Head Neck Surg 2006; 14:270–7.

8. McCurdy J. The Asian nose: augmentation rhinoplasty with L-shaped silicone implants. Facial Plast Surg 2002;18:245–52.

9. Raghavan U, Jones NS, Romo T III. Immediate autogenous cartilage grafts in rhinoplasty after alloplastic implant rejection. Arch Facial Plast Surg 2004;6:192–6.

10. Deva AK, Merten S, Chang L. Silicone in nasal augmentation rhinoplasty: a decade of clinical experience. Plast Reconstr Surg 1998;102:1230–7.

11. Conrad K, Gillman G. A 6-year experience with the use of expanded polytetrafluoroethylene in rhinoplasty. Plast Reconstr Surg 1998;101:1675–83.

12. Jin H, Lee J, Yeon JY. A multicenter evaluation of the safety of Gore-Tex as an implant in Asian rhinoplasty. Am J Rhinol 2006;20:615–9.

13. Romo T, Zoumalan R. Porous polyethylene implants in rhinoplasty: surgical techniques and long-term outcomes. Operat Tech Otolaryngol Head Neck Surg 2007;18:284–90.

14. Winkler AA, Soler ZM, Leong PL, et al. Complications associated with alloplastic implants in rhinoplasty. Arch Facial Plast Surg 2012;14(6):437–41 Published online Aug 29, 2012. Available at: http://www.archfacial.com/.

REFERENCES: TORIUMI

1. Toriumi DM, Pero CD. Asian rhinoplasty. Clin Plast Surg 2010;37:335–52.

2. Losquadro WD, Toriumi DM. Ethnic rhinoplasty. In: Nahai F, editor. The art of aesthetic surgery.

2nd edition. St Louis (MO): Quality Medical Publishing; 2011. p. 2101–47.

3. Toriumi DM. Discussion: use of autologous costal cartilage in Asian rhinoplasty. Plast Reconstr Surg 2012;130(6):1349–50.

4. Daniel RK. Diced cartilage grafts in rhinoplasty surgery: current techniques and applications. Plast Reconstr Surg 2008;122:1883–91.

5. Toriumi DM. Management of the middle nasal vault in rhinoplasty. Operat Tech Plast Reconstr Surg 1995;2(1):16–30.

6. Losquadro WD, Bared A, Toriumi DM. Correction of the retracted alar base. Facial Plast Surg 2012; 28(2):218–24.

7. Toriumi DM, Bared A. Revision of the surgically overshortened nose. Facial Plast Surg 2012;28(4): 407–16.

8. Gunter JP, Friedman RM. Lateral crural strut graft: technique and clinical applications in rhinoplasty. Plast Reconstr Surg 1997;99:943–55.

9. Toriumi DM. New concepts in nasal tip contouring. Arch Facial Plast Surg 2006;8:156–85.

10. Toriumi DM. Structure approach in rhinoplasty. Facial Plast Surg Clin North Am 2005;13: 93–113.

11. Angelos PC, Been MJ, Toriumi DM. Contemporary review of rhinoplasty. Arch Facial Plast Surg 2012; 14(4):238–47.

Lower Lid Blepharoplasty
Panel Discussion, Controversies, and Techniques

Shan Baker, MD[a],*, Keith LaFerriere, MD[b],*,
Wayne F. Larrabee Jr, MD[c,d],*

KEYWORDS

- Blepharoplasty • Cosmetic surgery • Surgery techniques • Orbital fat • Midface lift
- Aesthetic surgery • Oculoplastic surgery • Lower lid surgery • Eye rejuvenation surgery

---

Blepharoplasty Panel Discussion

Shan Baker, Keith LaFerriere, and Wayne Larrabee address questions for discussion and debate:

1. What is the most frequent displeasing effect you see when performing lower eyelid blepharoplasty?
2. What surgical approach do you most frequently use when performing lower eyelid blepharoplasty?
3. How much skin removal of the lower eyelids?
4. When performing lower lid blepharoplasty, what is your preferred method of managing pseudoherniated fat?
5. If you perform midface lifting during blepharoplasty, what approach do you use?
6. *Analysis*: Over the past 5 years, how has your technique or approach evolved or what is the most important thing you have learned in doing blepharoplasty?

 Keith LaFerriere presents videos of his blepharoplasty technique: video 1: Fat repositioning; video 2: transblepharoplasty, subperiosteal midface lift performed through a skin/muscle flap incision; and video 3: transtemporal subperiosteal approach to midface lift accompany this article at http://www.facialplastic.theclinics.com/

What is the most frequent displeasing effect you see when performing lower eyelid blepharoplasty?

BAKER

In my experience, the most common displeasing effect following lower eyelid blepharoplasty in patients operated on by other surgeons is lower eyelid retraction. In addition, in older patients with considerable loss of soft tissue volume of the midface, I usually see hollowing of the lower eyelids. This finding is presumably related to fat excision during blepharoplasty. I prefer fat preservation when performing lower eyelid blepharoplasty. My usual approach is advancement of fat

---

[a] Facial Plastic and Reconstructive Surgery, Department of Otolayngology, Head and Neck Surgery, University of Michigan, 19900 Haggerty Road, Livonia, MI 48152, USA; [b] Mercy Clinic - Facial Plastic Surgery, Springfield, MO, USA; [c] Larrabee Center for Facial Plastic Surgery, Seattle, WA, USA; [d] Department of Otolaryngology, Head and Neck Surgery, University of Washington, Seattle, WA, USA
* Corresponding authors.
E-mail addresses: Shanb@med.umich.edu (Baker); klaf1@sbcglobal.net (LaFerriere); larrabee@u.washington.edu (Larrabee)

Facial Plast Surg Clin N Am 22 (2014) 97–118
http://dx.doi.org/10.1016/j.fsc.2013.10.001
1064-7406/14/$ – see front matter © 2014 Elsevier Inc. All rights reserved.

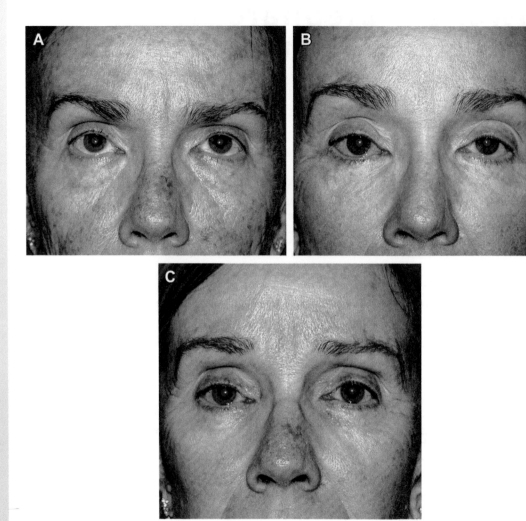

Fig. 1. LaFerriere. (*A*) Preoperative view. (*B*) Four weeks after skin/muscle flap blepharoplasty with lateral retinacular repositioning canthoplasty with persistent conjunctival edema right eye. (*C*) Three months postoperative image with resolution of the conjunctival edema and normal lid positioning. (*Courtesy of* Keith LaFerriere, MD, Springfield, MO. © Keith LaFerriere.)

and redundant septum over the inferior bony orbital rim into a subperiosteal space. The most common displeasing feature I identify in my personal patients is persistent visibility of pseudoherniated fat, particularly in the lateral compartments. In addition, in elderly patients with atrophic soft tissue cover in the periorbital region, the mobilized fat can sometimes produce a subtle contour fullness in the infraorbital zone.

LAFERRIERE

- *Conjunctival edema*, most commonly seen with a transconjunctival incision and fat repositioning: Steroid eye drops will usually aid in resolution, but rarely a small conjunctival unroofing is necessary (**Fig. 1**).

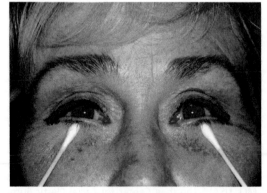

Fig. 2. LaFerriere. Patient 2 weeks after transconjunctival lower blepharoplasty with fat repositioning demonstrating restriction on upward mobility. This effect has always resolved over time, in my experience. (*Courtesy of* Keith LaFerriere, MD, Springfield, MO. © Keith LaFerriere.)

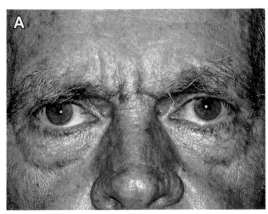
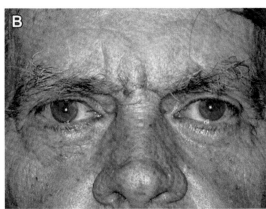

Fig. 3. LaFerriere. (*A*) Preoperative image. (*B*) Postoperative transconjunctival lower blepharoplasty with fat repositioning and lateral retinacular repositioning canthoplasty showing incomplete removal of the temporal fat pad. (*Courtesy of* Keith LaFerriere, MD, Springfield, MO. © Keith LaFerriere.)

- *Immobility of the lower eyelid* following a transconjunctival approach with fat repositioning: The lower lid should be able to be elevated to the superior limbus; but at times, there is restriction of the lid on the upward gaze. This effect almost always resolves with time and massage, but rarely triamcinolone 5 mg/mL injected into the middle lamella is needed. I have not seen a permanent problem with this (**Fig. 2**).
- *Incomplete excision of the temporal fat pad*, which can be seen as a lateral bulge: Meticulous removal of the temporal fat pad can greatly reduce this occurrence (**Fig. 3**).
- *Mild lateral rounding of the lid* with the skin/muscle technique: This effect can occur even if the flap is tacked laterally to the orbital rim. I think this is often related to the delayed return of function of the pretarsal orbicularis and usually resolves over time.
- *Epidermal inclusion cysts in the incision lines* secondary to suture tracts: These cysts are easy to correct but are a nuisance.

LARRABEE

There are several problems that may be accounted for after lower eyelid blepharoplasty, including dry eyes, hematoma formation, globe injury, infection, asymmetry, and lower eyelid malposition (ie, retraction, ectropion).[1] The techniques used in lower eyelid blepharoplasty have a major impact on the type of complication that may occur after surgery. For instance, the transconjunctival approach has a much lower rate of eyelid malposition[2]; the use of lateral canthal support significantly decreases the occurrence of scleral show and ectropion.[3] The most frequent long-term complication in skin muscle flap blepharoplasty is lower eyelid malposition, whereas persistent fat is most common in the transconjunctival approach. The most frequent problem I see after blepharoplasty is scleral edema, which almost always resolves spontaneously in a relatively short time. Of the 2 choices provided here, minor contour irregularities or scar visibility are most frequent. I am quite conservative and, therefore, the issue is usually persistent pseudoherniated fat, most commonly in the lateral fat pocket. If I use the pinch technique, I am focused on keeping the lateral scar subciliary because there is a tendency for it to move a little inferior in this area. Retraction of the lid is either caused by excess skin excision or scarring in the middle lamella together with preoperative lateral canthal laxity.[4] If a conservative approach is used during the skin-muscle flap technique, the risk decreases. It is uncommon to see eyelid retraction when performing a transconjunctival approach unless the middle lamella or, more specifically, the septum is damaged.

What surgical approach do you most frequently use when performing lower eyelid blepharoplasty?

BAKER

The most common approach I use in performing lower eyelid blepharoplasty is a fat-preservation blepharoplasty accomplished by first performing a skin pinch to precisely excise dermatochalasis. A skin muscle flap is dissected to the inferior bony orbital rim. The arcus marginalis is incised, and a subperiosteal pocket is dissected from beneath the tear-trough area laterally to the malar eminence. The septum is incised at the level of the inferior bony orbital rim near the medial canthus extending laterally to the attachment of the arcuate expansion. Redundant septum and fat are advanced as a composite flap into the subperiosteal space and secured in place. The septum is incised over the lateral compartment and fat is removed.

LAFERRIERE

The decision regarding the technical approach to lower blepharoplasty depends on the clinical findings at the time of consultation. The factors that enter into the choice of technique are multiple, including the sagittal bony orbital relationship to the cornea (vector anatomy), the extent of fat pseudoherniation, the amount of dermatochalasis present, the lid tone and position, and the presence of malar bags. Depending on the findings in each individual case, all of the aforementioned procedures are in my armamentarium.

The most frequent approach used is transconjunctival because it maintains the integrity of the orbicularis muscle, gives equal exposure to the to the fat pads as do the external techniques, and allows for a skin pinch and/or laser resurfacing to correct the dermatochalasis. If the skin excess can be eliminated by a pinch excision alone, carbon dioxide (CO_2) or erbium laser resurfacing is not used. If fine rhytids are present, or if skin excess is minimal, laser resurfacing alone is performed (**Fig. 4**). Skin excess and fine rhytids are treated with both skin pinch and laser resurfacing. This approach is also effective in patients who have very mild lid laxity because a canthoplasty can be avoided because the main supporting structures of the lid are maintained.

The skin/muscle external approach is used when there is extensive skin excess, festooning of the skin and orbicularis muscle, or malar bags (**Fig. 5**). Extending the skin/muscle flap in the suborbicularis oculi fat (SOOF) layer can improve malar bags in some instances (**Fig. 6**). Laser resurfacing can be used if fine rhytids are present.

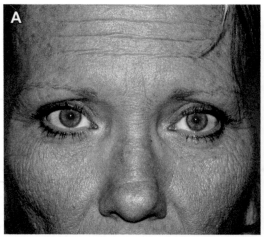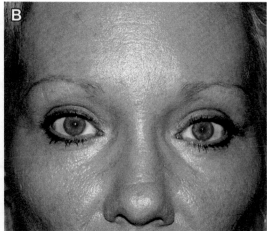

Fig. 4. LaFerriere. (*A*) Preoperative lower eyelid fine rhytids without significant dermatochalasis or fat pseudoherniation. (*B*) Postoperative CO_2 laser resurfacing without blepharoplasty demonstrating improvement of the fine lines. (*Courtesy of* Keith LaFerriere, MD, Springfield, MO. © Keith LaFerriere.)

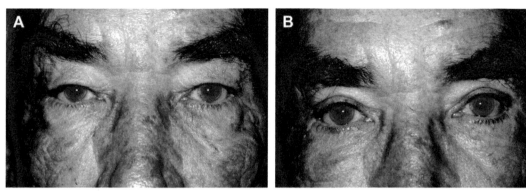

Fig. 5. LaFerriere. (*A*) Preoperative view of man with thick skin, significant dermatochalasis with fat pseudoherniation, and malar bags. (*B*) Postoperative extended skin/muscle lower blepharoplasty with fat repositioning and lateral retinacular repositioning canthoplasty, demonstrating the improvement in the dermatochalasis, fat pseudoherniation, and malar bags. (*Courtesy of* Keith LaFerriere, MD, Springfield, MO. © Keith LaFerriere.)

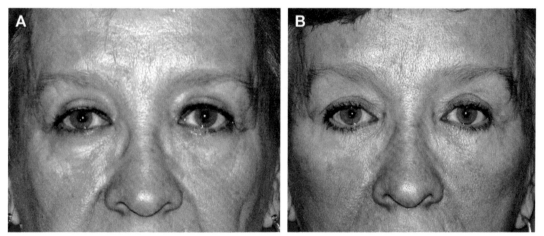

Fig. 6. LaFerriere. (*A*) Preoperative image of woman with dermatochalasis, fat pseudoherniation, and malar bags. (*B*) Postoperative extended skin/muscle flap over the SOOF to improve the dermatochalasis, fat pseudoherniation, and malar bags. (*Courtesy of* Keith LaFerriere, MD, Springfield, MO. © Keith LaFerriere.)

If there is no fat pseudoherniation present and predominantly skin excess exists without malar bags, a skin-flap lower blepharoplasty is very effective in these patients. If there is any form of nicotine use, this technique is contraindicated, as is laser resurfacing at the time of surgery. This approach is by far the least frequently used approach in my practice.

LARRABEE

I tailor my approach to the specific patient. The variables include a history of previous surgery; orbital anatomy, including the presence of a negative vector; skin texture and elasticity; lid tone; amount and location of pseudoherniated fat; presence of hypertrophic or lax orbicularis oculi muscle; and patient preferences. There are several techniques that may be used for lower eyelid blepharoplasty. These techniques include the skin-only approach, the skin-muscle flap, and the transconjunctival approach with or without skin excision. My most frequent approach is a transconjunctival blepharoplasty with a skin pinch. This technique allows for more controlled wound healing and, because the septum is left intact, has a lower tendency for scleral show or ectropion to develop.[5] Fat is managed as discussed later, with either excision or transposition. Resurfacing is performed in patients who desire to address their rhytids simultaneously. Frequently, these patients are undergoing a full-face laser resurfacing in addition to the treatment of the lower lid. I currently use both active and deep fx laser resurfacing with the Coherent system. TCA (Trichoroacetic Acid) peels (35%) and full phenol peels (88%) are still useful techniques for lower lid resurfacing in my patients. I still use a skin muscle flap blepharoplasty in special situations. The major indication for this technique is hypertrophic orbicularis muscle or an extremely lax orbicularis muscle where I wish to excise redundancy and tighten the lower lid. I will also use a skin muscle flap in secondary or revision cases where a skin muscle flap was used in the primary operations. In these cases, there are sometimes scar adhesions and other problems best addressed in the same plane of dissection.

How much skin removal of the lower eyelids?

BAKER

Dermatochalasis of the lower eyelids is treated with a skin pinch before developing a skin muscle flap. A standing cutaneous ridge is created 2 mm below the lash line using Brown-Adson forceps. Sufficient skin is incorporated into the standing cutaneous ridge to facilitate the removal of redundant skin. Before excising the ridge, the eyelid margin is examined to ensure that it is resting against the ophthalmic globe and there is no evidence of lid eversion or outward displacement of the punctum.

LAFERRIERE

With the transconjunctival approach, skin excision is relatively simple. I like to use hyaluronidase in the local anesthesia because it takes the swelling from local anesthesia out of the picture and the pinched skin stays elevated so accurate excision is possible. Using a Griffith-Brown or a Brown-Adson forceps, the skin is pinched approximately 2 mm below the lash line and the excess is gathered in the forceps, making sure that there is no distortion of the lower eyelid margin. This technique is how the amount of skin to be excised is determined.

With a skin/muscle flap technique, the incision is placed 3 to 4 mm below the lashes and beveled through the muscle to help preserve the pretarsal orbicularis function. When the flap is redraped, it is essential to make sure that the skin and muscle flap follows the contour of the underlying structure of the eyelid so that it is not tented because this will result in too much skin excised. With the patient's mouth open, the excess skin and preseptal orbicularis muscle can be safely removed. The skin-muscle flap is redraped in a predominantly superior direction with a slight lateral vector. There should be absolutely no tension on the suture line. It is important to tack the orbicularis and, hence, the flap to the lateral orbital rim to minimize lateral rounding of the lid.

With the skin flap approach, the skin is simply redraped, contoured to the underlying orbicularis muscle, and the excess excised. Because the orbicularis muscle is intact with this technique, I do not have patients open their mouth.

LARRABEE

Skin removal of the lower lids is relatively small and specific to the individual patient. With the pinch technique, the amount of skin is judged by using small forceps to pinch the excess skin after injection with local anesthetic and hyaluronidase. I use care to ensure the skin is draped into any lid concavities during this process. If patients are awake, I have them look up to help with this judgment. A conservative amount of skin is removed that causes no lid eversion. With a skin pinch excision, the same process is used but and the goal is to have the skin approximate with no sutures or tension. One removes more skin than it appears with a pinch, and a useful exercise is to stretch out the skin excised on a tongue blade after excision to measure the actual dimensions. In most cases, only a few millimeters need to be excised.

When performing lower lid blepharoplasty, what is your preferred method of managing pseudoherniated fat?

BAKER

My preferred method of managing pseudoherniated fat during lower eyelid blepharoplasty is mobilization of redundant septum and fat over the inferior bony orbital rim into a subperiosteal pocket. Pseudoherniated fat of the medial and central fat compartments is managed this way. However, I have not been successful managing pseudoherniated fat of the lateral compartment using this method.

Instead, I incise the septum overlying the lateral compartment and remove fat using a needle-tip electrocautery device.

LAFERRIERE

For the past 14 years, fat transposition over the orbital rim in a subperiosteal plane with direct excision of the temporal fat pad has been my preferred method of handling pseudoherniated fat in most patients. Following my patients for several years after the removal of pseudoherniated fat led me to the conclusion that, in the long-term, many developed a hollow-eyed appearance and often required fat transplantation for correction (**Fig. 7**). The result of fat repositioning is a smooth transition from the eyelid margin to the cheek, eliminating the tear trough and the appearance of circles under the eyes. The placement of the fat in the subperiosteal plane virtually eliminates the

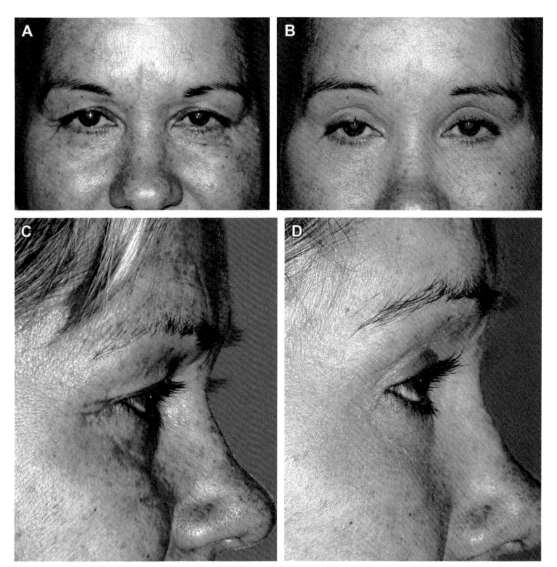

Fig. 7. LaFerriere. (*A, C*) Preoperative orbital hollowing following fat excision performed in a previous blepharoplasty. (*B, D*) One year after fat transplantation to the lower eyelids. (*Courtesy of* Keith LaFerriere, MD, Springfield, MO. © Keith LaFerriere.)

palpable lumps of fat that can occur with repositioning in the SOOF layer. Also, by releasing the orbicularis muscle from the orbital rim and arcus marginalis, the eyelid/cheek interface is elevated (**Figs. 8 and 9**).[1]

The absolute indication for fat transposition is in patients with negative vector anatomy, where in the sagittal plane the orbital rim lies posterior to the anterior extent of the cornea (**Figs. 10 and 11**). If fat is removed in these individuals, they have a very hollow appearance to the lower lids and often have an increase degree of scleral show. The same is true for big eyes, when the globe seems to protrude. Most patients with a neutral vector (whereby the orbital rim and the anterior plane of the cornea are on the same vertical line) will also have a nice result with fat repositioning. When the orbital rim is anterior to the anterior plane of the cornea (positive vector), I will remove the fat pads down to the level of the orbital rim because there is less chance of postoperative orbital hollowing.

Fat repositioning is easily performed through a transconjunctival or skin/muscle approach. With the transconjunctival incision, a 6-0 silk suture is placed through the retractor muscle and is

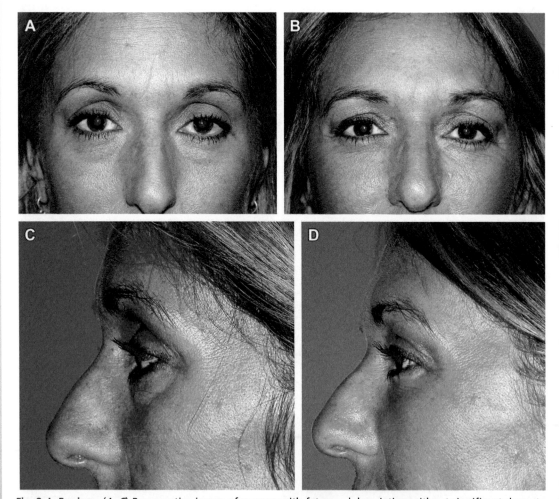

Fig. 8. LaFerriere. (*A, C*) Preoperative image of woman with fat pseudoherniation without significant dermatochalasis. (*B, D*) One-year postoperative image of transconjunctival lower blepharoplasty with fat repositioning. Note the more youthful distance from the eyelid margin to the cheek. (*Courtesy of* Keith LaFerriere, MD, Springfield, MO. © Keith LaFerriere.)

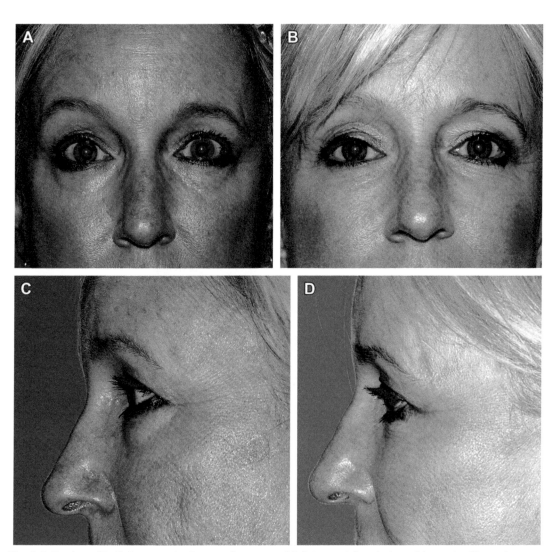

Fig. 9. LaFerriere. (*A, C*) Preoperative image of woman with fat pseudoherniation without significant dermato-chalasis. (*B, D*) One-year postoperative image of transconjunctival lower blepharoplasty with fat repositioning. Note the more youthful distance from the eyelid margin to the cheek. (*Courtesy of* Keith LaFerriere, MD, Springfield, MO. © Keith LaFerriere.)

clamped superiorly to the head drape to protect the cornea and put the orbital septum on stretch. When the skin/muscle exposure is used, the suture is placed through the pretarsal orbicularis and similarly clamped superiorly to the head drape. Keeping the orbital septum on stretch prevents overpull on the septum when the fat is being repositioned. In either instance, the periosteum is incised with cutting cautery at the orbital rim and

a subperiosteal pocket is dissected for several centimeters over the maxilla, taking care not to injure the infraorbital nerve. The orbital septum is incised at the arcus marginalis exposing the medial and middle fat pads. The fat pads are transposed with 3 transcutaneous sutures placed at the inferior extent of the subperiosteal pocket to secure the fat in the desired position. I have found that placing the medial fat pad and the

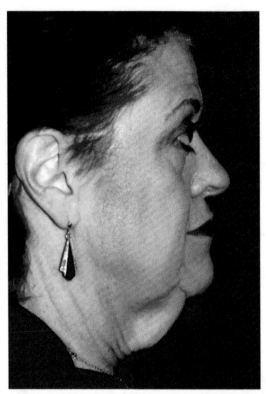

Fig. 10. LaFerriere. This patient demonstrates both negative vector anatomy, with the orbital rim significantly posterior to the anterior plane of the cornea, and big eyes. This type of anatomy is very dangerous if eyelid fat is removed rather than repositioned. (*Courtesy of* Keith LaFerriere, MD, Springfield, MO. © Keith LaFerriere.)

medial aspect of the middle (central) fat pad medial to the infraorbital nerve and the lateral portion of the middle fat pad lateral to the infraorbital nerve gives the best redraping of the fat over the orbital rim. The temporal fat pad is identified just above the Lockwood ligament and is removed because there is not enough mobility of this fat to be transposed. The sutures are taped to the cheek and removed at 1 week if laser resurfacing is not performed. With laser resurfacing, the sutures are tied through cut rubber tube bolsters (Video 1).

LARRABEE

Once more my management of the pseudoherniated fat depends on the anatomy and other variables specific to the patient. My general approach is to use some combination of excision and transposition. For example, if there is a small amount of lateral or medial fat, it is generally just excised to the level of the orbital rim. If there is a larger amount of middle fat, it is transposed depending on the local anatomy. Prominent orbital rims, negative vector, and tear-trough deformity represent situations whereby adding fullness to the infraorbital area is beneficial. I transpose fat from both the transconjunctival and skin muscle flap approaches. I almost never tighten the septum because middle lamella scarring is a prime cause of lid retraction. In certain cases whereby transposition of fat is insufficient, periorbital autologous lip injection or the use of hyaluronic acid fillers may be considered. This practice will be especially helpful in hollowed-out eyes or in patients with a major tear-trough deformity. The choice of hyaluronic acid fillers versus autologous fat is still an ongoing debate, and well-designed clinical trials will help us understand their relative merits.[6,7]

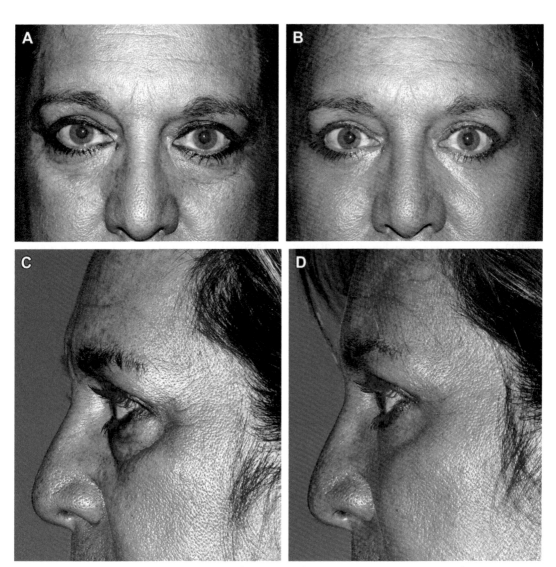

Fig. 11. LaFerriere. (*A, C*) Preoperative image of woman with negative vector anatomy and fat pseudohernia-tion. (*B, D*) One-year postoperative image of transconjunctival lower blepharoplasty with fat repositioning. Note the excellent lower lid contour without scleral show and the improved lid/cheek distance. (*Courtesy of Keith LaFerriere, MD, Springfield, MO. © Keith LaFerriere.*)

If you perform midface lifting during blepharoplasty, what approach do you use?

BAKER

When I perform midface lifting concomitant with lower eyelid blepharoplasty, I usually perform a subperiosteal midface dissection performed through a combined transtemporal and transoral approach. On occasion, I perform a deep-plane facelift to lift the soft tissues of the midface. In either case, I do not change my method of performing lower eyelid blepharoplasty.

LAFERRIERE

I have used all of these approaches to improve midface aging. Currently, the deep-plane technique is rarely used because, in my hands, the improvement in the midface has not been as good or as long lasting as the other procedures.

The main indication for a midface lift when performing a lower blepharoplasty is when the distance from the lower lid margin to the cheek junction is increased to the point that there is a significant paucity of soft tissue below the lid in spite of fat transposition. In addition, when the malar fat pad mounds against the melolabial fold, a midface lift can reposition the malar fat to a more pleasing position. I no longer reposition the orbital fat when doing a midface lift because the elevation of the cheek eliminates the need. In cases when a significant amount of pseudoherniated fat is present, the fat is removed down to the level of the orbital rim.

The best results for short- and long-term improvement in midface aging is the transorbital, subperiosteal technique (**Fig. 12**). The pull on the midface is directly vertical, and the release of the periosteum is complete, allowing for excellent midface repositioning and stable fixation. The procedure is entirely performed through the blepharoplasty incision and is less time consuming. Unfortunately, the recovery time is longer than with the transtemporal midface lift, sometimes taking as long as 6 weeks for the fullness in the lateral orbital area to subside. Lower eyelid malposition is a possibility if canthoplasty is not performed in the presence of lid laxity and/or if too much skin is removed from the lower eyelid.

The technique I like for the transblepharoplasty, subperiosteal midface lift[2] is performed through a skin/muscle flap incision. If lid laxity is diagnosed preoperatively, a canthoplasty or canthopexy must be performed at this time.

If fat pseudoherniation is present, the fat is removed down to the level of the infraorbital rim. Excess skin is excised as in a standard blepharoplasty at this time. No matter how much excess skin there seems to be at the end of the procedure, no more skin should be removed. Using a cutting cautery, the periosteum is incised along the orbital rim from as far medial as exposure will allow to laterally at the level of the lateral canthus and then laterally across the orbital rim at this level. This technique will allow for a periosteal flap to be raised superiorly from the level of the lateral canthus along the lateral orbital rim to be used later for fixation of the midface. The periosteum is then undermined over the face of the maxilla to the pyriform aperture and down to the level of

the ala and around to the lateral maxilla and zygomaticomaxillary junction. At this point, there is relatively little movement of the midface; but when the periosteum is completely released along the medial, inferior, and lateral extent of the subperiosteal dissection, an incredible amount of midface mobility is noted. The midface is then repositioned in a vertical direction; when the desired correction is achieved, the periosteum is sutured to the lateral orbital rim subperiosteal flap that was created earlier. Multiple sutures are used to secure the midface in the new, elevated position. Again, absolutely no more skin is removed from the lower lid despite the apparent excess because this ensures that there will not be an anterior lamellar deficit when the healing is complete. The incision is closed in the usual fashion (Video 2).

Because of the potential for a prolonged healing period, many patients will not opt for the transblepharoplasty, subperiosteal midface lift. For this reason, the transtemporal subperiosteal approach is the most commonly performed midface technique in my practice (**Fig. 13**). When I first started to do the temporal approach 18 years ago, the maxillary portion of the midface was accessed through the mouth and the temporal aspect was through an open incision combined with an open forehead/brow lift.[3] Much of the temporal dissection is relatively unchanged; but for the last 14 years, the midface is dissected through a transconjunctival incision. If steatoblepharon is present, the fat is removed down to the level of the infraorbital rim in the usual fashion. Cutting cautery is used to incise the periosteum along the infraorbital rim, and the subperiosteal dissection over the maxilla and medial zygoma is widely performed as in the transblepharoplasty approach described earlier. If a lower facelift is simultaneously performed, as is almost always the case, the preauricular incision is continued into the temporal area and angled slightly anterior. The temporal dissection proceeds on top of the superficial layer of the deep temporal fascia over the temporal line if an endoscopic forehead/brow lift is also being performed and subperiosteal over the lateral orbit and continued onto the zygoma and down to approximately 2 cm above the zygomatic arch. Care is taken to preserve the sentinel vein in this dissection. The dissection proceeds in the superior preauricular area to approximately 2 cm below the root of the zygomatic arch. An elevator is then used to dissect under the periosteum of the entire zygomatic arch, connecting the temporal dissection as one proceeds along the arch. Care must

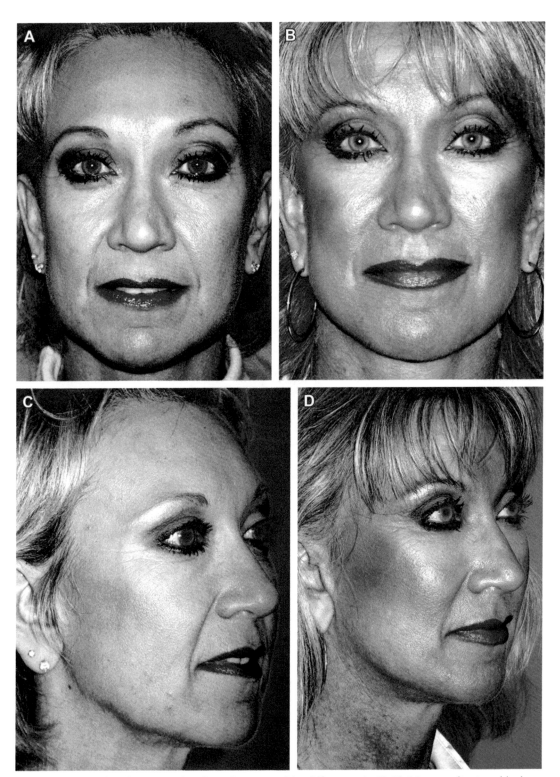

Fig. 12. LaFerriere. (*A, C*) Preoperative view of woman with midface ptosis; (*B, D*) 4.5 years after transblepharo-plasty, subperiosteal midface lift, and an extended SMAS rhytidoplasty with a corset platysmaplasty. Note the persistent elevation of the midface and the decreased distance from the lower eyelid to the cheek junction. This patient is shown in the movie. (*Courtesy of* Keith LaFerriere, MD, Springfield, MO. © Keith LaFerriere.)

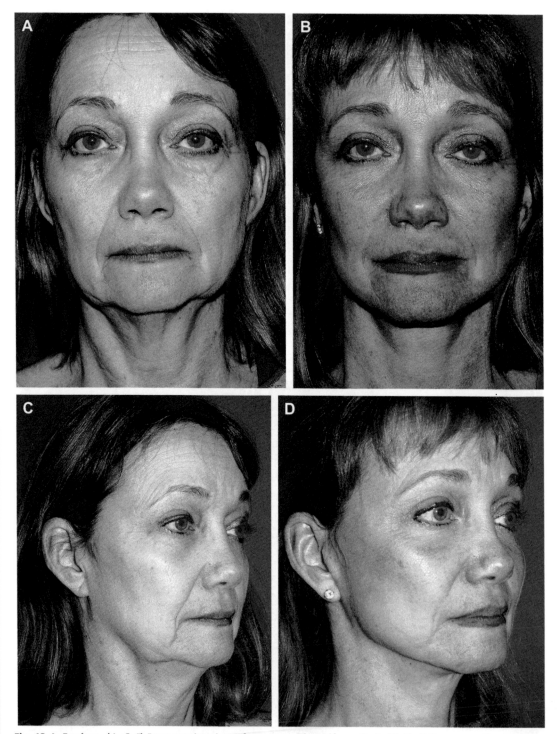

Fig. 13. LaFerriere. (*A, C, E*) Preoperative view of woman with midface ptosis. (*B, D, F*) One year after transtemporal, subperiosteal midface lift along with an extended SMAS rhytidoplasty with a corset platysmaplasty. (*Courtesy of* Keith LaFerriere, MD, Springfield, MO. © Keith LaFerriere.)

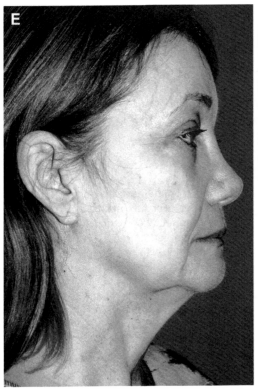

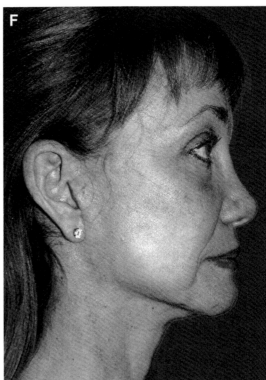

Fig. 13. LaFerriere. (*continued*)

be taken to dissect through the temporal fascia at least 1 cm above the arch to avoid injury to the frontal branch of the facial nerve. The remainder of the zygoma and the previously performed midface dissection can now be connected easily. The tissues are now elevated off of the temporomandibular joint fascia and proceeding anteriorly to about 2 cm below the arch onto the masseter muscle and over the fibers of the origin of the masseter muscle off of the inferior aspect of the body of the zygoma. This is necessary to get the desired mobility of the midface. With an assistant's finger protecting the lateral canthus, the periosteum along the inferior and lateral orbital rim is incised. Care must be taken not to disrupt the lateral canthus because this will create Asian-appearing eyes when the midface is lifted. The periosteum along the inferior and anterior aspect of the midface dissection is completely released; when this is accomplished, the midface is freely mobile in a superior and somewhat posterior direction. A 2-0 absorbable suture is passed through the periosteum on the undersurface of the flap at the level of the zygoma and sutured in as superior direction as possible to the temporal fascia, taking care not to tie this so tightly that it deforms the skin. This suture will hold the midface in the desired position until adhesion of the periosteum takes place. A second suture is placed through the fascia in the preauricular area about the level of the root of the zygoma and attached superiorly along the suture line to the temporal fascia. This placement gives about a 2-cm elevation of the lower midface and lower face for added improvement. This technique is shown very nicely in the movie (Video 3).

LARRABEE

Aging of the lower eyelid area is a multifactorial phenomenon, and some patients may benefit from surgery other than blepharoplasty. Endoscopic midface lifts can be combined with lower eyelid blepharoplasty to aid in decreasing the vertical length of the lower eyelid.[8] They may also help in retaining the shape and reducing tension on the lower eyelid over longer periods of time.[9] I perform both transtemporal midface lifts and deep-plane facelifts in combination with blepharoplasty. The transtemporal midface lift is used when there is primarily midface ptosis and little need to address jowls and neck laxity. It is also useful for secondary blepharoplasty procedures when there is the need to address lid retraction in combination with other problems of the aging lid. More commonly in a more complete facial rejuvenation, I combine a deep-plane lift with lower lid blepharoplasty to treat the neck, jowls, and midface simultaneously. It is possible to obtain a more vertical lift with the transtemporal approach, but the deep-plane lift also gives good improvement.

Analysis: Over the past 5 years, how has your technique or approach evolved or what is the most important thing you have learned in doing blepharoplasty?

BAKER

Over the last 5 years, I modified my approach to performing lower eyelid blepharoplasty. I find it difficult to properly mobilize orbital fat from the lateral compartment over the inferior bony orbital rim. I have attempted to tighten the septum in this area using sutures, thus reducing the pseudoherniation. However, my postoperative results using this approach have been disappointing. Frequently, patients would develop recurrence of the visible pseudoherniation. For this reason, I remove fat from the lateral compartment if patients present with pseudoherniation in this region of the orbit. I have also changed the way I advance fat over the inferior bony orbital rim from the central and medial compartments. I now incise the septum and advance redundant septum together with redundant orbital fat as a composite flap of tissue over the rim and into a dissected subperiosteal pocket. In my experience, advancing both the fat and septum creates a smoother and more uniform contour to the lower eyelid. Since adopting this technique, my long-term results are aesthetically more pleasing **(Fig. 14)**.

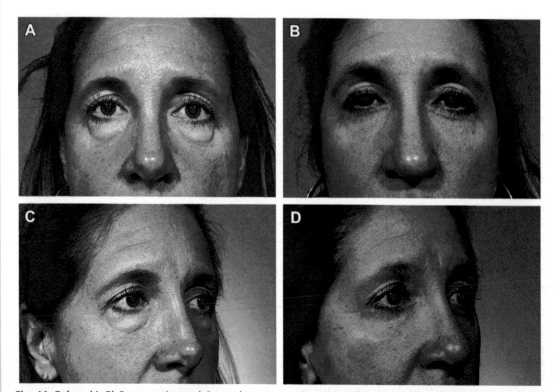

Fig. 14. Baker. (*A–D*) Preoperative and 6-month postoperative views of patient having fat-preservation lower eyelid blepharoplasty.

LAFERRIERE

I have not made major changes in my approach to lower eyelid blepharoplasty in the last 5 years, but a few things have evolved.

- Erbium laser with coagulation rather than CO_2 laser resurfacing is being used. I have had a few textural changes in the skin with the CO_2 laser and have noted quicker resolution of erythema and no textural problems with the erbium.
- Fewer patients are willing to undergo a midface lift, largely because of the economy.
- Hyaluronic acid fillers are used to touch-up postoperative irregularities. In patients that only have a mild tear trough, this can supplant a lower lid blepharoplasty.

- There is more use of the extended skin-muscle flap for mild malar bags. More extensive malar bags are treated with direct excision. Multiple treatments with a fractionated erbium laser have also proven helpful in some patients.
- There is increased use of fat transplantation for hollow orbits following previous fat excision blepharoplasties.

The most important thing I have learned doing lower blepharoplasty is that each set of eyelids is different and that no one technique fits all. One has to pay attention to the nuances and adjust the technique to fit the problem. Evaluating your patients postoperatively will be the single best way to improve your results.

LARRABEE

Early in my practice, as for most of my generation, I primarily performed skin muscle flap lower lid blepharoplasty. With the recognition of problems, mainly lid malposition, from middle lamella retraction, I changed and used transconjunctival approaches almost exclusively for many years. In the last 5 years, I have returned to the skin muscle flap lower lid blepharoplasty for specific cases as noted earlier. Although always aware of the importance of lid laxity, I have also become more proactive in performing canthopexy at the time of the

lower lid blepharoplasty in patients with lid laxity. I use a spectrum of canthopexy and canthoplasty procedures; but for preventative canthopexy in lids with minor laxity, I prefer the lateral retinaculum suspension suture in most situations. Finally, I have found fat transposition useful to aesthetically camouflage midface descent; but for numerous anatomic reasons, it is frequently suboptimal. I now recommend injections with hyaluronic acids or adipose tissue to add fullness over the rim, tear-trough area, and zone above the malar fat pad.

BAKER

Synopsis of my approach (with Video 4)

- A subciliary standing cutaneous ridge of skin of the lower eyelid is created with forceps and is excised (Fig. 15).[1,2]

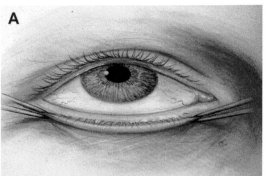
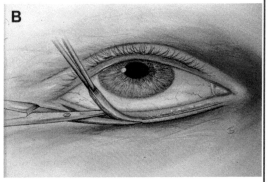

Fig. 15. Baker. (*A*) Standing cutaneous ridge is created immediately below the eyelashes. (*B*) Cutaneous ridge is excised exposing the orbicularis oculi. (*From* Baker SR. Orbital fat preservation in lower-lid blepharoplasty. Arch Facial Plast Surg 1999;1:34; with permission.)

- The eyelid margin is then retracted upward using suture suspension for protection of the cornea.
- The muscle is separated at the inferior border of the skin excision with microcautery electro-dissection preserving the pretarsal muscle (Fig. 16).

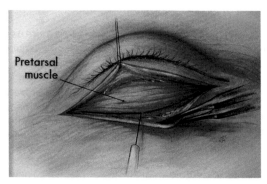

Fig. 16. Baker. An incision is made through the muscle preserving the pretarsal segment. (*From* Baker SR. Orbital fat preservation in lower-lid blepharoplasty. Arch Facial Plast Surg 1999;1:35; with permission.)

- A skin muscle flap is dissected inferiorly in a preseptal plane to the inferior bony orbital rim.
- The arcus marginalis is incised with electrocautery, and a subperiosteal dissection is performed with an elevator or with electrocautery.
- The dissection extends approximately 1.5 cm below the inferior bony orbital rim from near the medial canthus and laterally to the malar eminence exposing the SOOF located beneath the lateral half of the inferior aspect of the orbicularis muscle.

Surgical note: It is important to extend the dissection beneath the attachments of the levator labii superioris alaeque nasi to the upper part of the frontal process of the maxilla to ensure that the dissection extends beneath the nasojugal groove. Although the infraorbital nerve is not usually visualized, care is taken in the area of the nerve to prevent injury.

- At this stage, microcautery electro-dissection is used to incise the orbital septum at its junction with the arcus marginalis from the area of the medial canthus to the point of attachment of the arcuate expansion laterally (**Fig. 17**).

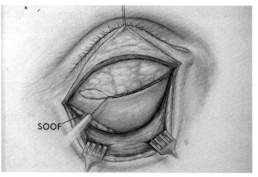

Fig. 17. Baker. Skin muscle flap is dissected to inferior bony orbital rim. Arcus marginalis is incised and a subperiosteal pocket is dissected 1.5 cm below inferior bony orbital rim. Orbital septum is divided from medial canthus to attachment of arcuate expansion to lateral third of bony rim. (*From* Baker SR. Orbital fat preservation in lower-lid blepharoplasty. Arch Facial Plast Surg 1999;1:35; with permission.)

Surgical note: This incision must be sufficient to allow the intraorbital fat to be freely mobilized over the inferior bony orbital rim with ease and without traction on the inferior oblique muscle.

- The redundant septum and pseudoherniated intraorbital fat are then advanced as a composite flap over the inferior bony orbital rim into the subperiosteal pocket.
- I secure the flap in place by using horizontal mattress 5-0 PDS (polydioxanone suture) sutures, which are inserted full thickness through cheek skin and the underlying soft tissue to incorporate the tissues of the advanced septum and fat.
- The mattress sutures are tied very loosely to prevent skin necrosis and scarring, which may occur from marked postoperative facial swelling. Usually 3 mattress sutures are necessary to maintain a uniform distribution within the subperiosteal space of the composite septal fat flap.

- On completion of mobilization, the skin muscle flap is redraped, the head is elevated, and the contour of the lower eyelid is assessed **(Fig. 18)**.

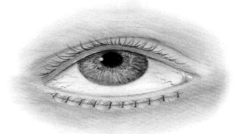

Fig. 18. Baker. Redundant fat and septum are advanced from medial and central compartments and secured in the subperiosteal pocket. Skin muscle flap is returned to the anatomic position, and the skin incision is sutured.

- In patients with pseudoherniated fat in the lateral eyelid compartment, an incision is made through the septum lateral and superior to the arcuate expansion. The fat is then teased out through the incision and removed using microcautery electro-dissection.

Adequate surgical exposure for fat advancement is more difficult through a transconjunctival approach than a transcutaneous approach and is reserved for patients with greater eyelid laxity.

- A transconjunctival incision is made with microcautery electro-dissection 3 to 4 mm from the inferior border of the tarsal plate.
- Electro-dissection continues through the lower eyelid retractors.
- The proximal conjunctival flap is then suspended upward over the cornea with a suture.
- With the eyelid on traction holding the conjunctival flap upward, electro-dissection continues in a preseptal plane down to the inferior bony orbital rim. This technique can be facilitated with blunt dissection using a cotton-tipped applicator.
- A Desmarrs retractor is inserted exposing the inferior bony orbital rim.
- The dissection then continues inferiorly over the rim just below the periosteum.

From this point forward, the dissection and advancement of redundant septum and fat is accomplished in a fashion identical to that described for the transcutaneous approach. The transconjunctival incision is closed with a few absorbable 6-0 sutures. A pinch-skin excision or resurfacing of the lower eyelids can be performed at the surgeon's discretion.

DISCUSSION

Hamra[3] has noted that in youth, the eyelid-cheek complex is a single mildly convex line on profile **(Fig. 19)**. Aging causes the descent of the globe and subsequent pseudoherniation of intraorbital fat, producing a double-convex lower eyelid contour on profile. Aging also causes the attenuation and descent of the orbicularis oculi and cheek fat. The inferior and lateral descent of these structures results in an increased distance from the lower lid margin to the inferior aspect of the orbicularis oculi, producing an orbit that appears deeper with a wider diameter.[3] This progressive ptosis and an attenuation of soft tissue coverage (skin and muscle) produces skeletonization of the entire orbital area and reveals the topographic contours of the inferior bony orbital rim.

Conventional lower lid blepharoplasty involves the removal of the intraorbital fat, which usually provides an adequate contour of the lid for several years. A sunken-eye appearance may develop,

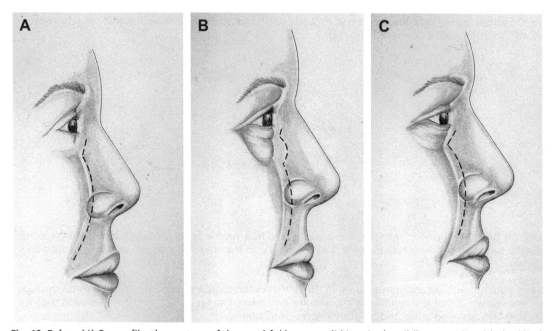

Fig. 19. Baker. (*A*) On profile, the contour of the youthful lower eyelid is a single mildly convex line (*dashed line*). (*B*) Aging causes pseudoherniation of intraorbital fat producing a double convex lower eyelid profile (*dashed line*). (*C*) Fat excision lower eyelid blepharoplasty may create a concave lower eyelid profile (*dashed line*) as patients age.

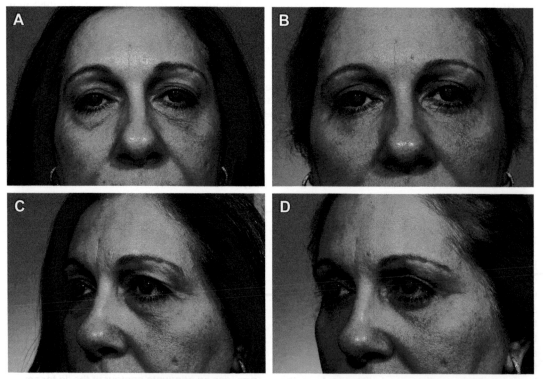

Fig. 20. Baker. (*A–D*) Preoperative and 6-month postoperative views of patient having fat-preservation lower eyelid blepharoplasty.

however, if excessive intraorbital fat is removed during lower lid blepharoplasty in patients with a visible nasojugal groove, deep-set eyes, or underdevelopment of the malar complexes. Even in younger patients without these manifestations, fat removal may cause a sunken-eye appearance as the SOOF, malar fat pad, and orbicularis oculi descend with age downward as a unit away from the orbital rim (see **Fig. 19**).[4] Over time, this descent and attenuation of soft tissue causes delineation of the bony orbital rim and a slight concavity just inferior to the rim. Removal of orbital fat only makes this hollow deeper, enhancing the tired look.[5] It seems reasonable to use the intraorbital fat to assist in effacing the inferior bony rim if clinically visible and, thereby, try to prevent or retard this manifestation of progressive aging. The long-term results of conventional blepharoplasty have not been studied, but I have observed patients having had blepharoplasty 10 to 20 years earlier. In this group of patients, skeletonization of the bony orbital rims appears more marked than in patients not having had blepharoplasty but who were of similar age and with similar skin and soft tissue coverage of the facial skeleton. Eder[5] has argued

that only a small percentage of younger patients have baggy eyelids caused by real excess of orbital fat. Increased orbital fat can also be found in rare cases of Graves disease.[5] These 2 conditions, according to Eder, represent the only true indications for fat removal.

The controversy surrounding my approach to lower eyelid blepharoplasty centers around the extent of dissection required for the technique. There tends to be more postoperative edema using fat-preservation procedures compared with fat excision blepharoplasty. There is a potential risk of restricting the movement of the inferior oblique muscle, although I have not encountered this phenomenon. I have also observed subtle but persistent visibility of the mobilized fat beneath the inferior bony orbital rim in some patients with marked atrophy of the soft tissues of the periorbital region. The greatest advantage of my approach is the prevention of the hollow eyelid observed in more elderly patients undergoing fat excision lower lid blepharoplasty. The advancement of intraorbital fat beneath the area of the nasojugal groove effectively eliminates the deformity that is associated with the aging lower eyelid **Fig. 20**).

SUPPLEMENTARY DATA

Supplementary data related to this article can be found online at http://dx.doi.org/10.1016/j.fsc.2013.10.001.

REFERENCES: BAKER

1. Baker SR. Orbital fat preservation in lower-lid blepharoplasty. Arch Facial Plast Surg 1999;1:33–7.
2. Fante RG, Baker SR. Fat-conserving aesthetic lower blepharoplasty. Ophthalmic Surg Lasers 2001;32(1):41–7.
3. Hamra ST. Arcus marginalis release and orbital fat preservation in midface rejuvenation. Plast Reconstr Surg 1995;96:354–62.
4. Hamra ST. Repositioning the orbicularis oculi muscle in the composite rhytidectomy. Plast Reconstr Surg 1992;90:14–22.
5. Eder H. Importance of fat conservation in lower blepharoplasty. Aesthetic Plast Surg 1997;21:168–74.

REFERENCES: LAFERRIERE

1. Couch SM, Buchanan HC, Holds JB. Orbicularis muscle position during blepharoplasty with fat repositioning. Arch Facial Plast Surg 2011;13(6):387–91.
2. Gunter JP, Hackney FL. A simplified transblepharoplasty subperiosteal cheek lift. Plast Reconstr Surg 1999;103(7):2029–35.
3. Nishioka GJ, LaFerriere KA, Renner GJ. Modified approach to the subperiosteal rhytidectomy. Plast Reconstr Surg 1996;97(7):1485–8.

REFERENCES: LARRABEE

1. Adamson PA, Constantinides MS. Complications of blepharoplasty. Facial Plast Surg Clin North Am 1995;3(2):211–21.
2. Mullins JB, Holds JB, Branham GH, et al. Complications of the transconjunctival approach: a review of 400 cases. Arch Otolaryngol Head Neck Surg 1997;123(4):385–8.
3. Honrado CP, Pastorek NJ. Long-term results of lower-lid suspension blepharoplasty a 30-year experience. Arch Facial Plast Surg 2004;6(3):150–4.
4. Hester TR Jr, Codner MA, McCord CD, et al. Evolution of technique of the direct transblepharoplasty approach for the correction of lower lid and midfacial aging: maximizing results and minimizing complications in a 5-year experience. Plast Reconstr Surg 2000;105(1):393–406.
5. Kim EM, Bucky LP. Power of the pinch: pinch lower lid blepharoplasty. Ann Plast Surg 2008; 60(5):532–7.
6. Yeh CC, Williams EF. Long-term results of autologous periorbital lipotransfer. Arch Facial Plast Surg 2011;13(4):252–8.
7. Stutman RL, Codner MA. Tear trough deformity: review of anatomy and treatment options. Aesthet Surg J 2012;32(4):426–40.
8. Marotta JC, Quatela VC. Lower eyelid aesthetics after endoscopic forehead midface-lift. Arch Facial Plast Surg 2008;10(4):267–72.
9. Villano ME, Leake DS, Jacono AD, et al. Effects of endoscopic forehead/midface-lift on lower eyelid tension. Arch Facial Plast Surg 2005;7(4): 227–30.

Midface Lift: Panel Discussion

Greg Keller, MD[a],*, Vito C. Quatela, MD[b],*,
Marcelo B. Antunes, MD[c],*, Jonathan M. Sykes, MD[d],*,
Christina K. Magill, MD[e],*, Rahul Seth, MD[f],*

KEYWORDS

- Midface lift • Panel discussion • Techniques

Midface Lift Panel Discussion

Greg Keller, MD with Rahul Seth, MD, Vito C. Quatela, MD with Marcelo B. Antunes, MD, and Jonathan M. Skyes, MD with Christina K. Magill, MD address questions for discussion and debate:

1. What is the most efficient dissection plane to perform midface lift?
2. What is the best incision/approach (preauricular, transtemporal, transoral)? Why?
3. What specific technique do you use? Why?
4. What is the best method/substance for adding volume to midface lifting?
5. In approaching the midface, how do you see the relationship of blepharoplasty versus fillers versus midface lifting?
6. Analysis: How has your procedure or approach evolved over the past 5 years? What have you learned, first-person experience, in doing this procedure?

 Dr Quatela and Dr Antunes provide 2 videos demonstrating the plane of dissection in midface lift (videos 1 and 2) along with 2 videos demonstrating placement of suspension sutures (videos 3 and 4)

What is the most efficient dissection plane to perform midface lift?

KELLER AND SETH

The midface lift can be performed in many dissection planes and efficient is a word that has many meanings.[1–12] So, it depends on what the surgeon wishes to do, how much effort that he/she wishes to expend, what his/her technical capabilities are, what the patient's signs of aging are, and what sort of result the patient expects.

There are 4 fat pads involved in midface lifting that can be repositioned:

1. Supraperiosteal fat pad, which contributes to the malar crescent and is bound to the periosteum and bone
2. Nasolabial or malar fat pad, which is held up by true ligaments to the malar eminence
3. Buccal fat pad, which is held up by false ligaments
4. Orbital fat, which can bulge anteriorly through the weakened orbital septum and over the orbital rim to the level of the fallen orbicularis retaining ligaments

---

[a] Keller Facial Plastic Surgery, David Geffen School of Medicine, University of California, Los Angeles, Santa Barbara, CA, USA; [b] Quatela Center for Plastic Surgery, 973 East Avenue, Suite 100, Rochester NY 14607, USA; [c] Antunes Center for Facial Plastic Surgery, Austin, TX, USA; [d] Facial Plastic Surgery, University of California-Davis Medical Center, 2521 Stockton Boulevard, Suite 7200, Sacramento, CA 95817, USA; [e] Division of Facial Plastic and Reconstructive Surgery, Department of Otolaryngology - Head and Neck Surgery, University of California-Davis, 2521 Stockton Boulevard, Suite 7200, Sacramento, CA 95817, USA; [f] Department of Otolaryngology- Head and Neck Surgery, Division of Facial Plastic and Reconstructive Surgery, University of California, San Francisco, San Francisco, CA, USA
* Corresponding authors.
E-mail addresses: faclft@aol.com (Keller); vquatela@quatela.com (Quatela); jonathan.sykes@ucdmc.ucdavis.edu (Sykes); christine.k.magill@gmail.com (Magill); rahul.seth@ucsf.edu (Seth)

Facial Plast Surg Clin N Am 22 (2014) 119–137
http://dx.doi.org/10.1016/j.fsc.2013.09.005

facialplastic.theclinics.com

Descent of these fat pads can be related to gravitational descent, stretching of the ligamentous attachments of these fat pads, and volume loss due to posterior retraction of the malar bone.

In addition, the superficial fascia/superficial musculoaponeurotic system (SMAS), deep fascia, and subcutaneous tissue fuse together and attach to bone at several locations in the midface. These occur at the orbit, the malar eminence, the massateric tendon/malar interface, nasal bone, zygomatic arch, frontal/zygomatic suture lines, etc). There are also ligamentous attachments of the SMAS that progress from bone to the skin of the midface (the malar ligaments, the orbicularis retaining ligament. Sagging of the skin and subcutaneous structures is related to the aging changes in these attachments. Another attachment related to malar edema is the "malar septum" extending from the arcus marginalis to the midface skin.

In addition, volume loss occurs in the face. This is present to a greater degree in the older patient. The skin of the midface is also not immune from the aging process. Both intrinsic and extrinsic causes of skin aging affect the midface.

To obtain a "best" natural appearance, deficiencies of aging related to these pathologies need to be addressed or camouflaged. Aging problems can be multiple and may vary individually or by age group. For instance, a 50 to 60-year-old woman will not have as much volume loss as a 75-year-old woman. Often a "smile test" is helpful to assess volume depletion of the midface. If the patient smiles and the fat pad ascends (meloplication) to fill out the cheek, it is likely that a surgical approach to lift the malar fat pad will work. If the fat pad does not add enough volume with the act of smiling, volume augmentation with filler or implants may be required.

At UCLA, we objectively evaluate our surgical approach based on the patient's pathology. We have looked at several indicators that help us to do this: the presence of an ogee curve; the distance from eyelashes to the optical bottom of the eyelid; orbital fat protrusion and degree of orbital fat "fall"; anterior projection of the malar eminence, and the presence of a negative or positive vector. While there are other subjective considerations, these indicators are useful in planning an approach. While we favor certain planes and approaches, we may use any or all of the planes that we list below.

For the younger patient, or the surgeon with limited technical capabilities, an "efficient approach" from a surgeon's perspective, may be to perform a subcutaneous face lift (with or without SMAS plication, such as a MACS or S-lift) and/or inject fat into the cheek to try to camouflage abnormalities. If there is a limited increase in distance

from the lashes to the apparent optical bottom of the eyelid, a decent ogee curve, and good anterior projection (all contributing to a "positive vector"), this may produce a happy patient and surgeon (and a short procedure). However, in many individuals, as the edema resolves and the fat disappears, the patient's preoperative and postoperative photos may not appear much different, except that the jowls and neck are resolved. If the only approach is to camouflage with filler in the setting of significant fallen fat pads, the patient may look artificially bloated ("puffer fish" abnormality) or the cheek may be filled, but the fallen malar pad may still protrude over the nasolabial fold ("rock in the sock" abnormality). In either case, the patient may exhibit an "artificial" appearance.

While many American authors are given credit for sub-SMAS or deep plane procedures, international surgeons are actually responsible for these more sophisticated approaches to the midface. Torg Skoog evolved the deep plane approach to the midface and Tessier, with his fellow, Mitz, explored and evolved the subperiosteal and "low" sub-SMAS procedures. Bosse and Papillon defined the malar retaining ligaments and sub-SMAS procedures to the midface that describe the facial nerve course. The procedures of Bosse and Papillon are, essentially, the "high SMAS" procedures that are used today. I had the privilege of meeting Bosse at an endoscopic meeting and discussing the implications of these procedures on the muscles of facial expression, which are significant and beyond the scope of this discussion. Reading of these authors is essential, should the surgeon wish to perform deeper procedures.

The "low SMAS" procedure involves a limited SMAS dissection plane below the zygomatic arch. Used alone, this approach, by itself, produces little effect on the midface unless it is carried over the malar eminence. It is often used with liporeinjection of the midface. The part of this procedure that is significant for the midface is that, with relaxation and fat reabsorption, a Nike "swoop" line can be produced as, over time, the midface sags over the tightened SMAS. A solution to this problem can be to partially support the midface with a percutaneous "meloplication" procedure of the fat pad or a subperiosteal elevation. For the surgeon with sufficient skill and the patient with a lesser degree of malar sag and shorter eyelid length, this can produce a nice result.

Another set of approach planes to the midface are the deep plane, suprafibromuscular, and "high SMAS" lifts. I group these together, as all of them release the malar ligaments and attachments. A Nike "swoop" line from midface relaxation is usually avoided, but the concavity of the ogee curve can be accentuated. All of these approaches, by freeing up the ligamentous

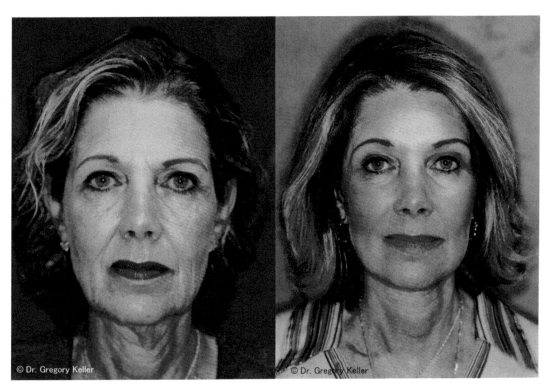

© Dr. Gregory Keller   © Dr. Gregory Keller

Fig. 1. Keller. Note the diminished distance from eyelash to bottom of the eyelid in this patient with a deep plane face lift and subperiosteal midface lift. (*Courtesy of* G. Keller, MD, Santa Barbara CA. © Gregory Keller.)

attachments of the midface, allow the malar fat pad to ascend, though this effect may be for a limited time. Combining these approaches with other midface lifting or augmentation techniques can produce a longer lasting result.

Another plane of dissection is the preperiosteal plane of dissection over the malar eminence. This plane of dissection extends under the suborbicularis oculi fat (SOOF) and over the deep fascia of the malar eminence. It is most commonly used from a blepharoplasty approach for orbital fat repositioning. The preperiosteal plane is also a "finger dissection" plane from a lateral and temporal face lift approach over the malar eminence and is used by some surgeons to elevate the malar area during a face lift.

The final plane of approach, and the one that we most often utilize, is the subperiosteal plane. This is the only plane that elevates the malar fat pad, the preperiosteal fat pad, and the SOOF. In

addition, the orbicularis muscle, the periosteum and overlying structures adherent to it, and the lip elevators can also be repositioned, if desired. A more extensive description of the technique follows. While a procedure involving a subperiosteal approach is not efficient from the surgeon's standpoint as it lengthens the procedure time, it is the most efficient approach to reposition fat pads, ligament, and muscle. Tessier described this procedure through a coronal approach and called it a "mask" lift, as it took the "mask" of the fallen face, and restored a youthful appearance (**Fig. 1**). When I viewed the results of this procedure, I was impressed that the pictures of Tessier, Psillakis and others using this approach were better than any others that I had seen. This procedure was invasive, and we began, in 1989 (procedure patented in 1991), to use an endoscope to reduce the edema associated with it.

QUATELA AND ANTUNES

The most efficient plane to elevate the midface is the subperiosteal plane. This plane can be elevated quickly with minimal bleeding. It is also a safe plane to avoid injury to nerves and the facial

mimetic musculature. The only nerves that are at risk are the frontal branch of the facial nerve and the maxillary division of the trigeminal nerve. The frontal branch can be avoided if the dissection is performed in the appropriate plane, elevating the periosteum without disruption. The maxillary nerve can be protected by palpation of the foramen and holding pressure at that point while the subperiosteal dissector elevates the midface above and below the exit of this nerve.

SYKES AND MAGILL

In general, the more superficial the dissection plane, the more efficient and secure the lift. Efficiency results from performing only the needed amount of dissection in order to achieve the desired result. In the forehead/brow, for example, the subcutaneous/suprafrontalis muscle dissection plane is more efficient than either the subgaleal or subperiosteal plane. The justification for performing further dissection, using a more distant incision, and developing a thicker flap is to hide the incision and preserve a vascular supply to the flap.

In the midface, the flap needs to be thick enough to camouflage suture irregularities (eg, dimpling), while allowing efficient undermining and elevation of the soft tissue envelope. The possible dissection planes for midface lifting include[1,2]:

1. Immediate subcutaneous plane
2. Sub-SMAS plane (superficial to the zygomatic musculature)
3. Preperiosteal plane
4. Subperiosteal plane (**Fig. 2**)

The subcutaneous plane has the greatest chance for contour irregularities, while the subperiosteal plane is the most inefficient, requiring the greatest release of soft tissues. The subcutaneous plane is the most efficient plane for elevation of the midface, but flap fixation can lead to contour irregularities of the facial skin.

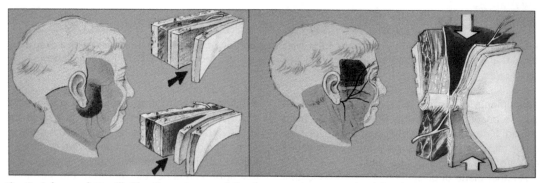

Fig. 2. Sykes and Magill. The tissue layers of the face are shown on the left: skin, subcutaneous issue, the superficial musculoaponeurotic system (SMAS) (investing fascia), the sub-SMAS plane (loose areolar tissue), and parotidomasseteric fascia (deep fascia). The image on the right demonstrates the fascial relationships at the level of the zygomatic arch. The frontal branch of the facial nerve travels in the temporoparietal fascia and is reflected laterally with the overlying subcutaneous tissue and skin. The deep layer of the temporal fascia is beneath the temporoparietal fascia and splits into a superficial layer and a deep layer. The superficial layer of the deep temporal fascia inserts onto the margin of the zygomatic arch and the deep layer of the deep temporal fascia inserts on the medial surface of the zygomatic arch. A fat pad is enveloped between the 2 layers of the deep temporal fascia. Beneath deep temporal fascia lies the deep temporal fat pad the temporalis muscle.

What is the best incision/approach (preauricular, transtemporal, transoral)? Why?

KELLER AND SETH

Generally, I prefer a temporal approach posterior to the hairline for lifting the midface. If the temporal incision is placed superior enough (close to the temporal line), an almost vertical direction of pull can be maintained. I will, on occasion, use an extended subciliary eyelid incision, in the face of severe temporal fascia scarring from previous procedures, though I can usually avoid this incision. An extended subciliary incision can produce an eyelid scar that needs to be covered with makeup, and can be associated with eyelid retraction and scleral show.

For positioning of an endotine in the proper position or for placing a malar implant, the intraoral incision is valuable. This incision gives the best access to the lower malar areas and the massateric tendon.

I will often use a transconjunctival incision to retroposition fat over the orbital rim, if orbital fat protrusion is a problem. Often, the orbital fat has protruded through a weakened septum, the globe has recessed, the SOOF fat has fallen, the orbicularis muscle has descended, and the malar fat pad has descended. Overall, this combination of aging effects produces the appearance of a "pot belly over fallen jeans." This set of anatomic problems can occur even in the younger individual. While all ethnic groups exhibit this "pot belly over fallen jeans" phenomena, many people of Middle Eastern and Asian descent manifest it at a relatively young age.

QUATELA AND ANTUNES

Over the course of the years, I have used transoral, transorbital, and transtemporal approaches to achieve midface elevation. In my opinion, the best incision/approach is the transtemporal.

The transtemporal approach, as the name illustrates, achieves midface elevation through a small temporal incision. The dissection starts separating the deep temporal fascia from the deep layer of the superficial fascia and from there to the subperiosteal plane. The forehead and the zygomatic arch are elevated subperiosteally, and this way, as previously mentioned, the frontal branch is protected. The dissection proceeds inferiorly, elevating the soft tissues of the midface from the maxilla. This approach has several advantages over the preauricular and transorbital approaches due to its vector of pull, increased lower lid support, and avoidance of lower lid malposition. In addition, this approach allows for a temporal lift simultaneously, which will elevate the lateral brow and avoid bunching of tissues in the temple. This way, the midface, lower lid, temples, and lateral brow are rejuvenated as a group, creating a more harmonious appearance. Initially, I combined this with a transoral approach to complete the dissection, but with more experience, I found this practice to be unnecessary, as I could get complete release of the midface from the temporal incision.

The preauricular approach can achieve midface elevation through a deep plane rhytidectomy dissection. In this approach, the SMAS layer is entered anterior to the frontal branch of the facial nerve and the dissection proceeds medially deep to the malar fat pad and superficial to the zygomaticus major muscle. After the zygomaticocutaneus ligaments are released, the malar fat pad can be elevated. The major advantage of the transtemporal approach over the preauricular approach is the vector of pull. The deep plane rhytidectomy has a more lateral vector, which is not optimal.

The transorbital approach also involves subperiosteal elevation of the midface soft tissue and its fixation to the deep temporalis fascia posterior to the orbital rim at a point just above the lateral canthus. The undermined skin-muscle flap elevated with the subciliary approach is then redraped and its excess removed. Following fixation and conservative excision of the lower lid skin, there is the need to create lower lid support, and this could be achieved with cathoplasty or a canthopexy, which can create several issues. Advocates for this technique claim that has the advantage of its dissection to avoid risk to branches of the facial nerve and create a vertical vector of pull. I don't think the frontal branch is under high risk with the transtemporal approach, since in over 1000 cases I only had one case of permanent paresis that occurred during a complex revision procedure. Moreover, this technique carries a higher risk of lower lid malposition and creates bunching of soft tissue and skin in the lateral orbital rim, sometimes creating an unnatural appearance. The transtemporal approach, on the other hand, will increase lower lid support and the concurrent temporal lift will avoid this lateral bunching.

SYKES AND MAGILL

The incision(s), approach, and fixation used to lift the midface are integrally related (ie, the incision used will affect the dissection plane and the method of flap fixation). There are several possible ways to approach the midface, including[3]:

1. Lateral temporal incision and approach

2. Transblepharoplasty approach with a transconjunctival or transcutaneous incision
3. Preauricular incision with a subcutaneous approach transitioning to a sub-SMAS plane

The advantages of a lateral temporal approach are the lateral vector of lift and the

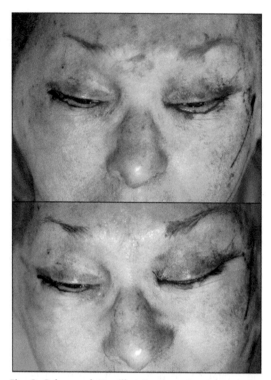

Fig. 3. Sykes and Magill. Intraoperative images of a transblepharoplasty approach to the midface. Transcutaneous incisions and lower blepharoplasties have been performed in the upper image. In the lower image, a left-sided midface lift has been performed. The left lid is tighter after fixation sutures.

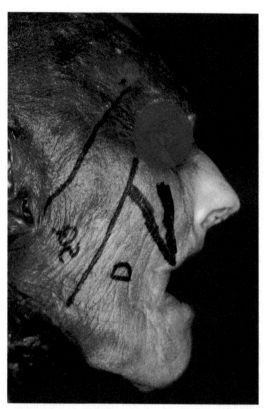

Fig. 4. Sykes and Magill. Landmarks for transition to the deep plane. The lateral mark demonstrates the approach to the midface in the subcutaneous plane. Note the more medial line drawn from the angle of the mandible to the right lateral canthus. The more medial line demarcates the transition to a deep plane of dissection. The deep plane of dissection is deep to the SMAS and superficial to the zygomaticus major and minor muscles, which have been marked out.

well-camouflaged incision. The transblepharoplasty approach provides good access to the midface, and a vertical vector of lift (**Fig. 3**). The level of the inferior orbital rim is the superior limit of the lifting vector with the transblepharoplasty approach.

I prefer the preauricular incision with a subcutaneous preauricular dissection plane transitioning to a sub-SMAS plane at a line which joins the mandibular angle with the lateral canthus (**Fig. 4**).

The reason for not initially dissecting in the sub-SMAS plane is that the superficial and deep fascia are fused in the immediate preauricular region. The midface flap is then fixated to the deep temporal fascia.

What specific technique do you use? Why?

KELLER AND SETH

I use almost every technique for addressing the midface that there is, depending on the pathology present. My favorite technique is the subperiosteal midface lift.

For the younger individual, filler substances are often the entry into cosmetic enhancement of the aging midface. Usually, these patients present in their 30s or 40s. There is not a great deal of pathology in these early midface patients, and they can

be filled conservatively, without producing the "bloated" look of a puffer fish.

As gravitational descent becomes more apparent, I most often use a subperiosteal midface lift with endotine fixation. Most of the patients in my practice exhibit gravitational descent as their primary problem as they approach and pass 50 years of age, particularly around and after the time of menopause. At this point, there is not usually a great deal of volume loss, and a natural facial rejuvenation can be obtained with surgery.

Through a temporal hairline incision, I dissect along the superficial layer of deep temporal fascia, pushing the temporoparietal fat pad and the innominate fascia superficially. I progress toward the zygomaticofrontal suture line until reaching the sentinel vein, which I cauterize with a bipolar if it is in the way of my dissection. I enter a subperiosteal plane at the lateral orbital rim and then dissect inferiorly over the malar eminence with a finger on the infraorbital nerve to protect it. Effort is also made to maintain the zygomaticofacial and zygomaticotemporal nerves. The dissection extends no further lateral than the medial third of the zygomatic arch, to avoid the temporal branch of the facial nerve. I may or may not use an endoscope, and the use of one is not mandatory.

At this point, I make a buccal gingival incision and carry the subperiosteal dissection upward to join the superior dissection. I also take down the fascial confluence of the malar periosteum and deep fascia of the massateric ligament, so that the periosteum can be freed and retracted upward. This is a similar approach to that of placing a malar/submalar implant. An endotine is placed through the gingivobuccal incisions and pulled superolaterally toward the temporal dissection. The endotine prongs enter the fascia and buccal fat pad, elevating these structures. The endotine is secured to the superficial layer of the deep temporal fascia.

The endotine fixation has a number of advantages. It elevates all of the major cheek fat pads, increases cheek projection, and restores the ogee curve. By using this fixation, it is not necessary to elevate the periosteum past the medial one-third over the zygomatic arch. This avoids exposure to the temporal branch of the facial nerve.

Another procedure that I use is to "meloplicate" the cheek fat pad. This technique uses a Gore-Tex suture to suspend the malar fat pad to the temporal fascia, and is described in our previous publications. It can be performed by a percutaneous technique. I reserve this procedure for patients who wish to undergo a less extensive or less costly procedure.

QUATELA AND ANTUNES

 Dr Quatela and Dr Antunes provide 2 videos demonstrating the plane of dissection in midface lift (videos 1 and 2) along with 2 videos demonstrating placement of suspension sutures (videos 3 and 4)

My preferred technique is the transtemporal subperiosteal approach for all the reasons described above (optimal vector of pull, increased support of the lower eyelid, and concurrent elevation of the temple). Every time I perform a subperiosteal midface elevation, I perform brow repositioning and a lower blepharoplasty at the same time.

In further detail, I start by marking the temporal incision approximately 1 cm behind the hairline at the superior aspect of the temporalis muscle, and this incision continues for 3 cm inferolaterally. I have the patient contract his/her temporalis muscle to see where the temporal line is, and I make sure that the starting point is 1.5 to 2 cm inferior to the superior temporal line, otherwise the suspension sutures into the deep temporal fascia will be difficult to place. When making the incision, I bevel the scalpel parallel to the hair follicles, preserving them to achieve maximal scar camouflage, as transecting the hair follicles results in a few millimeters of permanent alopecia. The medial incisions for brow suspension begin a few millimeters behind the hairline centered over the lateral canthus and extend posteriorly for 2 cm.

The temporal incision is carried down through the superficial temporal fascia to the deep temporal fascia. A dissector is used to elevate the superficial temporal fascia and overlying tissue off the deep temporal fascia to the temporal line. The dissection continues superiorly in a subperiosteal plane and ends at the level of the occiput. This ensures that the elevated forehead and lateral temporal tissues will redrape and not bunch anteriorly once suspended. Inferior to the incision, dissection on top of the deep temporal fascia is performed blindly for 2 to 3 cm. Anteriorly, this elevation requires lysis of the fascia at the temporal line, and subperiosteal dissection is continued to the supraorbital rim. The arcus marginalis often can be released from lateral to within 1 cm to the notch of the supraorbital neurovascular bundle. Bimanual dissection often is helpful, and the hand placed on the surface of the skin helps prevent injury to the orbit with inferior dissection. Laterally, the conjoint tendon is dissected bluntly. If this fascial condensation is not released adequately, elevation of the lateral brow will be incomplete during suspension.

With inferior temporal dissection, I take extra care in the region of Pitanguy's line. In this area there are multiple bridging veins that penetrate the plane of dissection perpendicularly in the region of the frontal branch of the facial nerve are encountered during this dissection (**Fig. 5**). I am also very careful in the temporal region, because forceful dissection may result in penetration

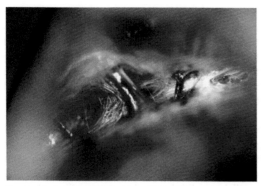

Fig. 5. Quatela and Antunes. Endoscopic view of the zygomaticofacial vein (sentinel vein), which estimates the course of the frontal branch of the facial nerve.

through the deep temporal fascia, which would expose the infratemporal fat pad, and even minimal trauma can result in reduction of its volume with temporal wasting postoperatively. With further inferior dissection, I encounter the zygomatic arch. At the level of the deep temporal fascia split, the intermediate temporal fat is encountered, being safe to dissect within this fat pad. However, I prefer to elevate the intermediate fat pad up and dissect on top of the deep temporal fascia. I believe that elevating all these tissues helps provide an additional cuff of tissue to insulate the frontal branch from thermal or mechanical trauma.

I preserve an area of 1 cm lateral to the lateral canthus to prevent permanent canthal distortion postoperatively. Even though initially the eye may look pulled, the preservation of the canthal insertion ensures that the eye will return to normal after a few weeks. Over the zygomatic arch, the periosteum over the entire superior aspect is exposed, and it is incised at the anterior aspect of the arch. The zygomaticofacial foramen often is encountered and the neurovascular structures kept intact, as this is an important landmark for later suspension of the midface. Subperiosteal dissection continues posteriorly at the superior edge of the zygomatic arch to within 1 cm of the external auditory canal. Once the edge is exposed, the periosteum over the zygomatic arch is released. This subperiosteal dissection is continued medially over the infraorbital rim to the nose in a blind fashion. Bimanual dissection is required with the dissector passed between the index finger that protects the globe and the thumb positioned over the infraorbital nerve. The periosteal dissector is then passed subperiosteally starting at the body of the zygoma directed toward the pyriform aperture, inferior to the infraorbital nerve. This accomplishes dissection over the face of the maxilla and with a superior sweeping motion releases all tissue inferior the

infraorbital nerve. I avoid violating the buccal mucosa. Some surgeons perform an incision there, but I find it unnecessary. The only time I make an incision is when there is excessive bleeding in the midface and that incision allows for drainage. Subsequentially, the tendinous attachments at the lateral aspect of the maxilla are lysed with the down-biting dissector, and the masseteric tendon just inferior to the inferior aspect of the zygomatic arch is cut with a downward motion. The flap is dissected inferiorly below the masseteric aponeurosis just on top of the belly of the masseter to approximately 1 cm superior to the gonial angle. The medial subperiosteal midface dissection pocket and lateral submasseteric aponeurosis pocket are connected with a sweeping finger dissection from the medial to lateral pocket breaking the last few fascial attachments at the lateral aspect of the maxilla. This dissection accomplishes a complete release of the midface as well as the tissues laterally to the external auditory canal and inferiorly to the level of the gonial angle. This ensures free mobility of the midface, malar fat pad, and SOOF (see Videos 1 and 2 for the demonstration of the plane of dissection online at).

I suspend the midface and temples with 5 sutures. The first one is from the released periosteum just lateral to the zygomaticofacial foramen to the deep temporal fascia at a vector superior and slightly lateral. The second suspension suture is placed posterior and superior to Pitanguy's line in the flap and back to the deep temporal fascia. These 2 sutures will create the midface suspension. In addition, I place 3 suspension sutures at the anterior skin edge through the superficial temporal fascia, suspending it to the deep temporal fascia posterosuperiorly in the region of the temporal line. These 3 sutures are the reason the placement of the lateral incision is so important, because placement of the incision too high will prevent the ability to suspend the excess skin of the temporal region that bunches after elevation of the midface (see Videos 3 and 4 for the placement of suspension sutures, online at). With the midface lift, even if a full endoscopic forehead lift is not performed, a lateral temporal lift with release of the arcus marginalis and conjoint tendon is done and prevents bunching of skin in the lateral temporal region. After the midface and temples are suspended, the forehead elevation is performed. Two removable screws are placed into the holes drilled through the medial incisions, the forehead is then retracted posteriorly until its leading edge rests against the screw, and a staple is placed just behind the screw. This most anterior staple sits behind the screws and prevents the forehead flap from gravitating inferiorly.

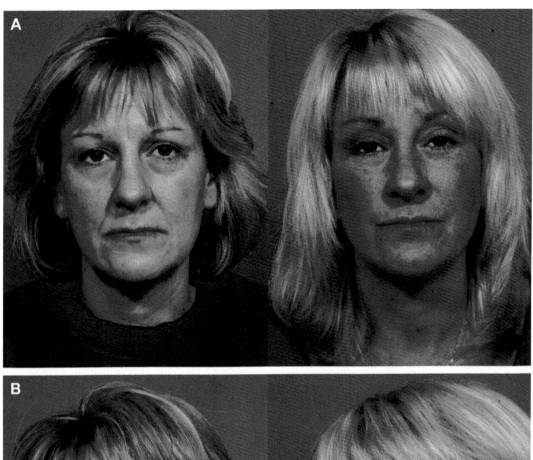

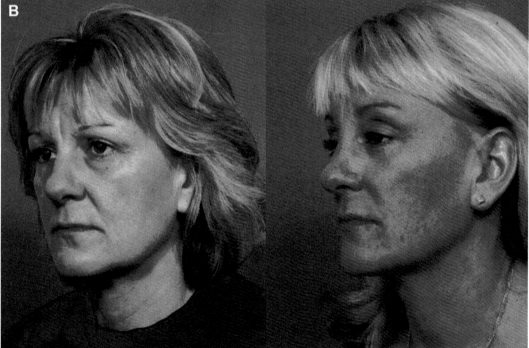

Fig. 6. Quatela and Antunes. Before and after frontal (*A*) and three-quarter (*B*) views following an endoscopic midface lift. Note the correction of the double contour deformity of the lower eyelid with padding of the inferior orbital rim, elevation of the midfacial fat pads, and improvement in the jowling.

The lateral temporal incisions are closed with sutures. **Fig. 6** illustrates the result after a midface lift.

SYKES AND MAGILL

In most individuals, I use the preauricular approach to the midface. The preauricular approach offers good camouflage for incisions, a wide lateral vector arch for lift, and reliable fixation. The preauricular incision is made with a standard retrotragal (or tragal top) incision in females, and a pretragal incision in males. The incision is carried to a level just inferior to the tragus (if midface lifting is performed alone) and is carried around the ear lobule if lower face lifting is also being performed. Sharp dissection is used in the preauricular subcutaneous plane. At a line joining the mandibular angle and the lateral canthus, the sub-SMAS plane is entered. After the plane is entered with sharp dissection, blunt dissection can be accomplished to extend the deep sub-SMAS plane (**Fig. 7**).[4,5] The mandibulocutaneous and zygomaticocutaneous ligaments are then lysed to mobilize the midfacial flap (**Fig. 8**).

In the temporal region, a pretrichial or sideburn splitting incision is used to expose the deep temporal fascia. Back dissection deep to the temporoparietal fascia exposes the dense deep temporal fascia (**Fig. 9**). This is a rigid structure that is immobile and provides a good

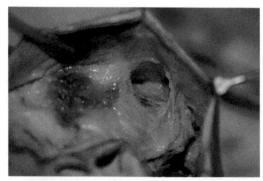

Fig. 8. Sykes and Magill. Right face of a cadaver following the dissection of a subcutaneous and sub-SMAS flap. The deep plane can be seen in focus, and the subcutaneous dissection proximally is out of focus. It is important to lyse all zygomaticocutaneous and mandibulocutaneous ligaments.

foundation for fixation of the facial flap. After full mobility of the facial flap and exposure of the deep temporal fascia, fixation sutures may be placed. These are accomplished from the edge of the SMAS in a running locking fashion to the deep temporal fascia. Additional individual sutures from the malar fat pad to the deep temporal fascia are also performed. Suture fixation is accomplished with 2–0 monofilament absorbable sutures.

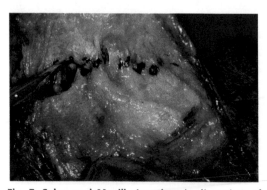

Fig. 7. Sykes and Magill. A cadaveric dissection of the left face demonstrating the transition from the subcutaneous to the deep plane. A flap has been developed in the subcutaneous plane. Scissors held at a 90° angle to the tissues are used to enter the deep plane. This transition is made distal to a line drawn from the angle of the mandible to the lateral canthus.

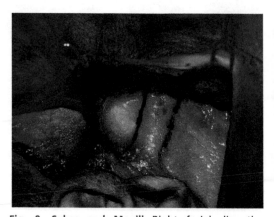

Fig. 9. Sykes and Magill. Right facial dissection demonstrating the deep temporal fascia on the left side of the image with the temporoparietal fascia elevated with the skin flap. The zygomatic arch has been marked out and the dissection plane below this is in the subcutaneous plane. The traversing line marked out delineates the expected course of the frontal branch of the facial nerve.

What is the best method/substance for adding volume to midface lifting?

KELLER AND SETH

For the congenitally narrow face in the patient that does not wish major bony distraction surgery, the best solution is probably a malar/submalar implant. That being said, I almost never use malar implants as a solution for facial aging.

If I see a patient who is not ready for a surgical procedure, I regard liporeinjection as an excellent volumizer. However, there are several problems with fat injections that have caused me to back away from the technique, in recent years (I've performed liporeinjection since 1982). One is that the procedure, as a "non-surgical" procedure has a very rare incidence of blindness. While I would not let that stop me from personally having liporeinjection, I find that many patients, once informed of this risk, opt out of liporeinjection. While many patients might accept the risk of blindness with a surgical procedure such as blepharoplasty, these same patients associate fillers with no risks of significance and are not willing to accept a risk of blindness for a less invasive procedure.

Currently, my "go to" filler for the midface is a combination of platelet rich plasma (PRP) and hyaluronic acid (HA). I first inject the HA to the areas of concern, and then inject the PRP, which is activated with calcium chloride or gluconate. The HA acts as a scaffold for the PRP. The amount of HA injected is not enough to provide a meaningful fill without the PRP. I use a blunt needle for the injection, and there is rarely any bruising.

Sclafani has provided evidence-based research that the PRP activates a cellular process with 5 effects:

1. PRP activates unipotent stem cells.
2. PRP promotes angiogenesis, which improves the color and texture of the skin.
3. PRP promotes activation of fibroblasts, which secrete collagen and thicken the skin.
4. PRP promotes activation of adipocytes within the skin, which encourages volume filling and repair.
5. PRP provides a fill which lasts approximately 18 months.

Our experience has been that patients without a great deal of sagging do quite well with this procedure, which we most often use as a prelude to a midface lift.

In the office, and for the patient wishing a "quick solution," commercially available fillers suffice. These include HAs, sculptra, and Radiesse. These are covered more completely by other authors.

Another surgical method of providing volume to the midface (in addition to midface lifting and meloplication) is orbital fat transposition. Doubtless, this technique is covered by another author of this journal. It is worth mentioning, however, that with the arcus marginalis release and the transposition of fat over the malar eminence, the orbicularis re-establishes itself at a more superior level and some of the orbicularis "sag" is reduced. As a result, the eyelash-to-bottom-of-eyelid distance becomes shorter.

QUATELA AND ANTUNES

The most popular way of adding volume to the midface is by autologous fat transfer or synthetic fillers. My personal preference is to volumize the midface with fat grafting; however, this involves a procedure in the operating room. If the patient has reservations regarding going to the operating room or cannot afford any downtime, I offer synthetic fillers. Also, I often use fillers in addition the midface lift in the postoperative period when patients have severe loss of facial volume. In very few occasions, in patients that require a large volume replacement, I place a submalar implant and add more volume with fillers and fat as needed.

Fat has been described as the being the ideal filler because it is biocompatible, lacks toxicity,

has a low cost, a very low incidence of complications, and is a renewable resource.[1] Autologous fat transfer for facial rejuvenation is not a new idea. Since its first successful report, over a century ago,[2] multiple studies reported variable results with fat transfer. There has been great disparity on the reported results in regard to graft survival and long-term outcomes, with volume retention ranging from 10% to 90%.[3–6] It is important to observe that the vast majority of these data comes from subjective analysis of patients' photographs. Very few studies actually report objective measurements of volume retention using magnetic resonance imaging and three-dimensional photography[7,8] with long-term success rates in those studies ranging from 30% to 45% of the initial injected volume. My impression is that patients usually retain about 60% of the injected volume at 1 year after injection. In my experience, patients retain that volume even after many years providing they do not have significant weight loss. The physiology of adipocytes explains why some fat graft volume loss happens due to tenuous blood supply at the recipient site, and until angiogenesis is complete, the cells are nourished by diffusion.[9] This led to the conclusion that the larger the graft, the greater would be the degree of resorption. Additionally, inflammatory infiltrates that surrounded the fat grafts would contribute to cell loss and subsequently volume loss. This highlights the importance of atraumatic tissue handling during harvest and injection and empha-sizes the importance of fat processing to eliminate fatty acids, blood products, and cellular debris that would exacerbate the local inflammatory response. My preference is to use a syringe-assisted liposuction is the least traumatic way to obtain the grafts; however, there is a great deal of controversy in methods used to prepare and inject the fat. These include the mixture of insulin, growth factors and β-blocker washes among others.[10–13] I do not use these products, and just prepare the fat by removing all the oil from the syringe, washing it, and subsequently centrifuging it to further remove the oil and blood. This step cannot be overemphasized for the reasons mentioned above. Injection is usually performed with blunt cannulas into the soft tissues. Several passages are made with the cannulas to disperse the fat within the tissue, enhancing the surface area between the cells and surrounding tissues. Because my preferred technique of midface lifting involves subperiosteal elevation, I do not perform fat transfer at the same time of surgery.

Of the commercially available ones, poly-L-lactic acid (PLLA) is the best for volumizing the malar regions. This product provides the most clinically noticeable volume, with the least amount of product used. Administration involves a depot injection of product on the malar eminence and in the regions of greatest volume loss followed by deep subcutaneous fanning with cross-hatching, creating a layering effect of product. This technique helps to evenly distribute the filler throughout the cheek region. Filling the submalar region can significantly improve the drawn ap-pearance associated with hollowness in this re-gion, which is often seen with significant weight loss. Patient counseling is especially important when using PLLA due to its delayed effect. More-over, most patients usually require more than 1 treatment, with 3 treatments spaced 6 weeks be-tween injections constituting the most common clinical scenario. In some cases, several additional treatments may be necessary over a 4- to 6-month period to obtain optimal volume. Collagen produc-tion usually starts in 6 to 8 weeks[14] following injec-tion, and continue to form for up to 9 to 12 months after the last treatment.[15] The volumetric benefits lasts about 2 to 3 years.[16] Meanwhile, PLLA parti-cles start to be reabsorbed around 6 months and disappear by 9 months.[17]

SYKES AND MAGILL

Although permanent alloplast implants are used by many surgeons, I prefer autologous fat to augment the soft tissues of the midface and pro-vide volume to this area. Alloplasts provide per-manent augmentation, but the issues related to this surgery can create long-lasting soft tissue complications. Fat augmentation has the disad-vantage of being impermanent in its effect. How-ever, fat can be placed in more areas and is more titratable. In order to be effective, allo-plasts are typically placed over bone and require bony fixation. Fat can be placed in various layers of the face and has the advantage of creating radial, three-dimensional soft tissue augmentation.[6]

When placing fat in addition to static lifting, I prefer to inject the fat after the lifting procedure is completed and the incisions are closed. By performing the fat augmentation as a final step, I believe I have the most control over volume augmentation and a better appreciation for the areas that need to be filled.

In approaching the midface, how do you see the relationship of blepharoplasty versus fillers versus midface lifting?

KELLER AND SETH

All of these procedures have their place. Orbital fat transposition blepharoplasty, as mentioned above, can be useful in the younger individual and, in Middle Eastern and Asian patients to elevate the orbicularis muscle (via an arcus marginalis release) and to fill a portion of the midface with orbital fat.

Fillers are usually used, in my practice, for the younger patient or the patient reluctant to commit to surgery or transcutaneous meloplication. The fillers are usually performed in the office with either local or topical anesthesia.

If a smile test is positive, and the patient is willing to undergo a minor procedure under local anesthesia, I will perform a transcutaneous meloplication. If the patient is willing to undergo an IV anesthesia, then a subperiosteal midface lift is preferred. At times, the midface correction may obviate the need for a lower blepharoplasty fat correction. Lifting the malar fat pad and SOOF may lift the "fallen jeans" over the "pot belly" of fallen fat.

Malar bags, due to orbicularis retaining ligament relaxation, preperiosteal fat, edema, and excess eyelid skin remain a challenge. My best results involve combining blepharoplasty with a temporal subperiosteal midface lift.

If a patient has a genetically narrow midface, then I might recommend malar or submalar implants.

QUATELA AND ANTUNES

The midface lift, blepharoplasty and fillers are intimately related when it comes to midfacial rejuvenation. I consider these 3 modalities as part of a spectrum to create a youthful midface. One of the most important goals in approaching the midface is the effacement of the lower lid-cheek junction and restoration of the contour of the cheek and malar eminence. Sometimes, these goals can be achieved with fillers or fat transfer alone or in combination with blepharoplasty and sometimes a midface lift is required to achieve those goals. It is important that the understands the aging process and how it affects these structures so he/she can better counsel the patient on which would be the best approach. Aging changes in 1 anatomical region will have an impact the neighboring areas; the midface ages together with the lower lid in the same manner that the brow ages with the upper eyelids.

In patients with loss of facial volume and minimal soft tissue ptosis, synthetic fillers or autologous fat transfer can improve the lid-cheek junction and create a rounder and smoother cheek. I usually use a combination of HA and PLLA for the tear trough and malar eminence, respectively. The HA is placed deeply, at the level of the orbital rim while the PLLA is placed as described above. If the patient is willing to go the operating room, I prefer fat transfer, which I perform in isolation or in combination with other procedures. However, I rarely perform fat transfer for the midface and infraorbital rim at the same time I do a subperiosteal midface lift. If decision is made on a lift, my preference is to allow the soft tissues to settle after the lift and decide on the need of volume augmentation at a later time. I have been surprised that more often than not, soft tissue reposition alone will abbreviate the need for volume replacement.

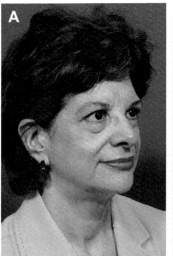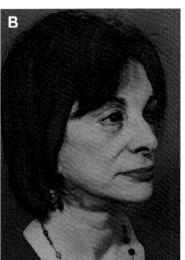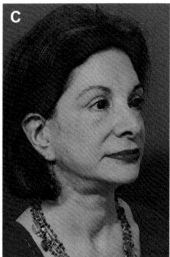

Fig. 10. Quatela and Antunes. Photos of patient with severe midfacial ptosis and loss of facial volume submitted to a midface lift. The patient initially underwent a midface lift (*A*) before and (*B*) after 1 year postoperatively. Subsequently this patient underwent autologous fat transfer (*C*).

In some patients with mild to moderate midfacial soft tissue ptosis and exposure of the orbital rim, I often perform either a midface lift or a lower blepharoplasty. I have a discussion about the difference in downtime and recovery period for both procedures and educate the patient on what each procedure can achieve. If decision is made to proceed with a lower blepharoplasty alone, I usually perform a fat transposition to pad the orbital rim, especially if the patient has a negative vector. This procedure alone will fill the lid-cheek junction but will not address the cheek or suffice in patients with more midfacial soft tissue ptosis.

In patients with significant exposure of the inferior orbital rim and midfacial soft tissues ptosis, my preference is to perform a midface lift. It is

important to realize that the patients who will benefit more from the midface lift are also the same ones who are in most need of volume augmentation. This is explained to the patient preoperatively and I add volume as described above. Moreover, I perform a lower blepharoplasty in every midface lift without exceptions. The extent of the lower blepharoplasty is usually a simple skin excision with or without transconjunctival fat removal. The skin excision can be more aggressive than usual due to the fact that midface suspension will increase the tension in the lower lid and decrease the risk of lid retraction.[18] **Fig. 10** illustrates this point demonstrating a patient with severe midfacial ptosis and loss of facial volume who underwent a midface lift and a subsequent session of autologous fat transfer.

SYKES AND MAGILL

I rarely perform midface lifting through a blepharoplasty approach. It is safer to remove lower eyelid skin when midface lifting is performed in conjunction with lower blepharoplasty. The midface lift creates a foundation for the lower eyelid and a supportive sling to the lid. Volume augmentation of the midface, whether with "off-the-shelf" fillers or autologous fat, also supports the lower eyelid and increases safety for lower eyelid skin excision.

The decision to perform surgical lifting and lower blepharoplasty versus soft tissue filling is based on the individual diagnosis of the patient and on the patient's preference for surgical versus noninvasive enhancement. Clearly, aesthetic surgeons have realized that filling the lower eyelid-cheek junction is as important as lifting of the soft tissue structures.[7] Often, a combination of these techniques is required to maximize facial appearance and rejuvenate the midface.

Analysis: over the past 5 years, how has your technique evolved or what is the most important thing you have learned doing midface lifts?

KELLER AND SETH

The best available procedure for restoring the midface remains the subperiosteal midface lift, as first described by Tessier (mask lift). Psillakis noted that the procedure avoided injuries to the temporal branch of the facial nerve if the subperiosteal dissection extended no further laterally than the medial one-third of the zygomatic arch. Fixation of the malar fat pad was not as easy with this limited dissection until the endotine fixation device avoided the problems of "cheese wiring" that occurred with sutures. In the late 1980s and early 90s, we used a "loop" fixation of Gore-Tex delivered transcutaneous with the subperiosteal dissection. This has remained a "backup" fixation to this day.

For the patient that does not wish to commit to a surgical solution to the midface, other procedures are available, but do not address many of the structural ramifications of aging. The subperiosteal midface lift reliably addresses many of these, and

restores the structures of the face to their natural position.

As an aside, our approach to the aging face is a restorative one. While there are many articles that define the "ideal" dimensions of the face, we do not necessarily try to duplicate these dimensions and proportions in our aging face corrections. Changing an aging face patient's facial dimensions from their previous youthful features has different ramifications than changing dimensions in younger patients. Most aging face patients that I see in my practice prefer a "natural" look that restores their own youthful beauty. That being said, no rule is without an exception (**Figs. 11–13**).

A midface lift (sometimes called an "endoscopic face lift") may be performed as a sole procedure in the younger patient, or as a revision in a patient who has had a face lift without correction of midface ptosis. However, I most

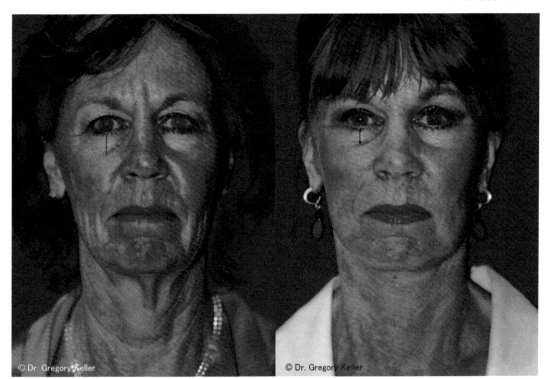

Fig. 11. Keller. Preoperative (*red arrows*) and postoperative (*blue arrows*) height of the lower lid, as measured from the lid margin to the lid-cheek junction. There is a significant reduction in the height of the lower lid following a midface lift. (*Courtesy of* G. Keller, MD, Santa Barbara CA. © Gregory Keller.)

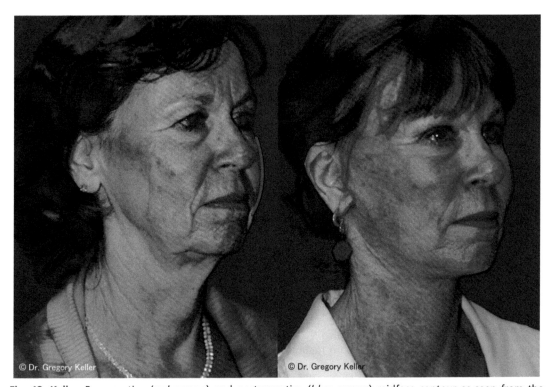

Fig. 12. Keller. Preoperative (*red arrows*) and postoperative (*blue arrows*) midface contour as seen from the three-quarters oblique view. Note the restoration of the ogee curve following midface lift. (*Courtesy of* G. Keller, MD, Santa Barbara CA. © Gregory Keller.)

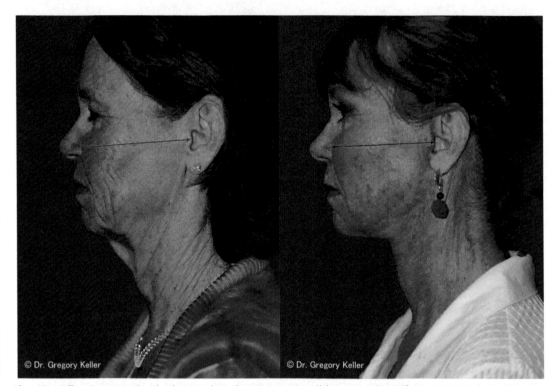

Fig. 13. Keller. Preoperative (*red arrows*) and postoperative (*blue arrows*) midface projection measurement demonstrating a modest but noticeable increase following a midface lift. (*Courtesy of* G. Keller, MD, Santa Barbara CA. © Gregory Keller.)

often perform a midface lift in association with a face lift procedure that addresses the facial ligament sagging, first described by Skoog, Bosse, and Papillon and subsequently by Furnas. As noted above, the midface lift procedure often is a part of the overall aging face correction.

For the younger patient, or the patient that does not wish to invest the financial resources or wishes to avoid surgery, fillers, the percutaneous midface lift, and more limited facial procedures may represent a reasonable "compromise" solution to the midface. Because of the rare instance of blindness, many of these patients, when informed of this complication, decide against liporeinjection. For many of these, an HA combined with PRP injection has offered an acceptable alternative.

QUATELA AND ANTUNES

In my opinion, perhaps the biggest advancement in the rejuvenation of the midface over the last decade was our better understanding of the aging changes that occur in the area. In addition to the changes in the skin envelope, significant changes occur in the soft tissues and underlying craniofacial skeleton. This concept has reinforced my feelings that not only the ptotic midface should be repositioned but also volumetrically augmented to achieve a more natural result.

Over the past 5 years, I have not changed my surgical technique significantly. I perform less orbicularis myotomies to elevate the brow further, because this leads to prolonged supraorbital and upper eyelid edema. When I suspend the midface, there is no tension on the sutures, since the elevation is a result of an adequate release of the soft tissue envelope. My suspension is also less aggressive, which avoids lateral canthal distortion. I also routinely preserve the sentinel vein and the other bridging veins, as this will decrease the skin and subcutaneous engorgement on the temple and forehead in the postoperative period. All this minor adjustments that I learn over the last 20 years of midface lifting made big improvements in achieving a natural and long-lasting outcome.

SYKES AND MAGILL

Patient satisfaction from midface rejuvenation is based on a combination of factors. These include careful patient selection, individualized diagnosis, and meticulous execution. I am selective in which patients I offer midface lifting to. Specifically, many patients are less-than-ideal candidates for midface lifting secondary to the fact that their expectations include resolution of fine midfacial skin rhytids and near-total effacement of the melolabial folds. These improvements are typically not achievable. Additionally, I realize that three-dimensional volume enhancement of the face is as important

as surgical lifting. The dominant focus on volume restoration of the face in order to achieve a more youthful appearance has augmented, and in some cases replaced, midface lifting. In order to achieve ideal midfacial rejuvenation, a combination of these techniques is usually necessary (**Fig. 14**).

SUPPLEMENTARY DATA

Supplementary data related to this article can be found online at http://dx.doi.org/10.1016/j.fsc.2013.09.005.

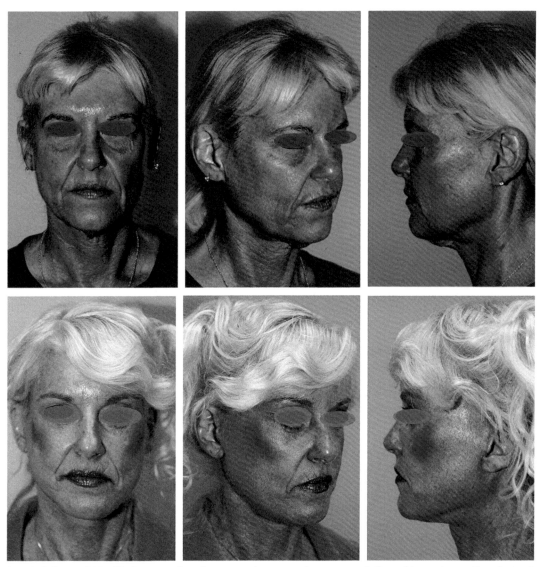

Fig. 14. Sykes and Magill. Preoperative photos are shown on the top row, followed by postoperative photos in the bottom row. The patient has undergone bilateral upper and lower blepharoplasties, a lateral temporal brow lift, a midface lift, and neck lift. Combined procedures were used to give the patient an optimal cosmetic result.

REFERENCES: KELLER & SETH

1. Jorge MP, editor. Deep facelifting techniques. New York: Thieme; 1994. This is a "must read" for every surgeon serious about facelifting.
2. Pessa JE, Garza JR. The malar septum: the anatomic basis of malar mounds and malar edema. Aesthetic Surg J 1997;17(1):11–7.
3. Keller GS, Namazie A, Blackwell K, et al. Elevation of the malar fat pad with a percutaneous technique. Arch Facial Plast Surg 2002; 4(1):20–5.
4. Heffelfinger R, Blackwell K, Rawnsley J, et al. A simplified approach to midface aging. Arch Facial Plast Surg 2007;9(1):48–55.
5. Keller GS, Kang RS. Biostimulation of our own cells for skin rejuvenation. Oral presentation. AAFPRS rejuvenation of the Aging Face. San Diego (CA), January 2012.
6. Kang R, Lee M, Seth R, et al. Outcomes of the subperiosteal midface lift. Presented: AAFPRS Spring Meeting. Orlando (FL), April 2013. Submitted for publication: JAMA Facial Plastic Surgery.
7. Kahn DM, Shaw RB. Overview of current thoughts on facial volume and aging. Facial Plast Surg 2010;26(5):350–5.
8. Yaremchuk MJ, Kahn DM. Periorbital skeletal augmentation to improve blepharoplasty and midfacial results. Plast Reconstr Surg 2009;124(6):2151–60.
9. Newman J. Safety and efficacy of midface-lifts with an absorbable soft tissue suspension device. Arch Facial Plast Surg 2006;8(4):245–51.
10. Punthakee X, Mashkevich G, Keller GS. Rejuvenation of the lower lid and periocular area from above. Facial Plast Surg 2010;26(3):232–8.
11. Keller GS, Cray J. Suprafibromuscular facelifting with periosteal suspension of the superficial musculoaponeurotic system and fat pad of Bichat rotation. Tightening the net. Arch Otolaryngol Head Neck Surg 1996;122(4):377–84.
12. Andretto Amodeo C, Kang R, Keller GS. The suborbicularis oculi fat (SOOF) and the fascial planes: has everything already been explained? Presented: AAFPRS fall meeting. September 2012. Accepted for publication: JAMA Facial Plastic Surgery.

REFERENCES: QUATELA & ANTUNES

1. Coleman SR. Structural fat grafts: the ideal filler? Clin Plast Surg 2001;28(1):111–9.
2. Neuber F. Fett transplantation. Chir Kong Verhandl 1893;1:66–8.
3. Ersek RA. Transplantation of purified autologous fat: a three year follow-up is disappointing. Plast Reconstr Surg 1991;87(2):219–27.
4. Fulton JE, Suarez M, Silverton K, et al. Small volume fat transfer. Dermatol Surg 1998;24(8):857–65.
5. Fournier PF. Fat grafting: my technique. Dermatol Surg 2000;26(12):1117–28.
6. Coleman SR. Long-term survival of fat transplants: controlled demonstrations. Aesthetic Plast Surg 1995;19(5):421–5.
7. Hörl HW, Feller AM, Biemer E. Technique for liposuction fat reimplantation and long-term volume evaluation by magnetic resonance imaging. Ann Plast Surg 1991;26(3):248–58.
8. Meier JD, Glasgold RA, Glasgold MJ. Autologous fat grafting: long-term evidence of its efficacy in midfacial rejuvenation. Arch Facial Plast Surg 2009;11(1):24–8.
9. Peer LA. Loss of weight and volume in human fat grafts. Plast Reconstr Surg 1950;5:217–30.
10. Moscona R, Shoshani O, Lichtig H, et al. Viability of adipose tissue injected and treated by different methods: an experimental study in the rat. Ann Plast Surg 1994;33:500–6.
11. Yuksel E, Weinfeld AB, Cleek R, et al. Increased free fat-graft survival with the long-term, local delivery of insulin, insulin-like growth factor-I, and basic fibroblast growth factor by PLGA/PEG microspheres. Plast Reconstr Surg 2000;105:1712–20.
12. Ayhan M, Senen D, Adanali G, et al. Use of beta blockers for increasing survival of free fat grafts. Aesthetic Plast Surg 2001;25:338–42.
13. Nguyen A, Pasyk KA, Bouvier TN, et al. Comparative study of survival of autologous adipose tissue taken and transplanted by different techniques. Plast Reconstr Surg 1990;85:378–86.
14. Lacombe V. Sculptra: a stimulatory filler. Facial Plast Surg 2009;25:95–9.
15. Gogolewski S, Jovanovic M, Perren SM, et al. Tissue response and in vivo degradation of selected polyhydroxyacids: polylactides (PLA), poly(3-hydroxybutyrate) (PHB), and poly(3-hydroxybutyrate-co-3-hydroxyvalerate) (PHB/VA). J Biomed Mater Res 1993;27:1135–48.
16. Mest DR, Humble GM. Duration of correction for human immunodeficiency virus-associated lipoatrophy after retreatment with injectable poly-L-lactic acid. Aesthetic Plast Surg 2009; 33:654–6.
17. Lowe NJ. Optimizing poly-L-lactic acid use. J Cosmet Laser Ther 2008;10:43–6.
18. Villano ME, Leake DS, Jacono AD, et al. Effects of endoscopic forehead/midface-lift on lower eyelid tension. Arch Facial Plast Surg 2005;7(4): 227–30.

REFERENCES: SYKES & MAGILL

1. Tessier P. Lifting facial sous-perioste. Ann Chir Plast Esthet 1989;34:193 [in French].
2. Mendelson BC, Muzaffar AR, Adams WP. Surgical anatomy of the mid-cheek and malar mounds. Plast Reconstr Surg 2002;100(3):885–96.
3. Freeman MS. Rejuvenation of the midface. Facial Plast Surg 2003;19(2):223–36.
4. Hamra ST. The deep-plane rhytidectomy. Plast Reconstr Surg 1990;86(1):53–61.
5. Sykes JM, Liang J, Kim JE. Contemporary deep plane rhytidectomy. Facial Plast Surg 2011;27(1):124–32.
6. Stallworth CL, Wang TD. Fat grafting of the midface. Facial Plast Surg 2010;26(5):369–75.
7. Hester TR, Codner MA, McCord CD, et al. Evolution of technique of the direct transblepharoplasty approach for the correction of lower lid and midfacial aging: maximizing results and minimizing complications in a 5-year experience. Plast Reconstr Surg 2000;105(1):393–406.

Distraction Osteogenesis

James Sidman, MD[a],*, Sherard Austin Tatum, MD[b],*

KEYWORDS

- Distraction osteogenesis • Orthognathic surgery • Distraction osseogenesis • Maxillofacial surgery
- Craniofacial surgery • Facial skeletal surgery

Distraction Osteogenesis (DO) Panel Discussion

James Sidman, MD and Sherard A. Tatum, MD address questions for discussion and debate:

1. Is neonatal DO better than lip-tongue adhesion or tracheotomy for micrognathic airway compromise?
2. What role does DO have in adult orthognathic surgery situations?
3. In monobloc and Le Fort III procedures, are internal or external devices preferable?
4. What role does DO play in craniofacial microsomia?
5. Is endoscopic DO better than open procedures for synostosis management?
6. Analysis: how has your technique changed or evolved over the past 5 years and what has doing this technique taught you?

Is neonatal DO better than lip-tongue adhesion or micrognathic airway compromise?

SIDMAN

Tongue-lip adhesion (TLA) will certainly work in neonates with minimal airway compromise. There is however the "elephant in the room" with TLA, and that is the issue of swallowing after the surgery. Most studies looking at this carefully are showing very high rates of gastrostomy, even in nonsyndromic children. Our own papers show a very low rate of needing gastrostomy with distraction osteogenesis (DO) during infancy.

We also feel that nasal airway ("trumpet") is underutilized in most institutions in the management of micrognathic children. If indeed the trumpet works, then TLA is not necessary as they both accomplish the same thing. Either the trumpet or TLA really only works in the less severely affected children.

The last item to address is the issue of isolated micrognathia. We have found very few children with micrognathia who have airway obstruction based on the micrognathia and do not also have full blown Pierre Robin sequence (RS) with cleft palate, glossoptosis, and micrognathia. When we are referred airway obstructed babies without the triad of Pierre Robin, then invariably the airway issue is caused by something other than

---

Disclosures: None.

[a] ENT and Facial Plastic Surgery, Children's Hospitals and Clinics of Minnesota, University of Minnesota Medical School, 2530 Chicago Avenue S, Suite 450, Minneapolis, MN 55404, USA; [b] Cleft and Craniofacial Center, Division of Facial Plastic Surgery, Upstate Medical University, 750 E. Adams Street, Syracuse, NY 13210, USA
* Corresponding authors.
E-mail addresses: sidma001@umn.edu (Sidman); tatums@upstate.edu (Tatum)

micrognathia and DO is almost never the appropriate treatment.

In summary, we have little use for TLA as we would use either a nasal trumpet, or proceed to DO of the mandible. The significant deleterious effects of TLA on swallowing should not be discounted, and seems to be almost universal.

TATUM

MDO for airway compromise in the neonate/infant micrognathic patient was introduced in 1999.[1] Until then positioning, special feeding techniques, temporary pharyngeal airways, TLA, and tracheotomy were the main options. Similar controversy existed then among those options. The addition of MDO has not diminished the controversy. There has been no definitive comparative study published that clearly shows the superiority of one method over the others. This conundrum exists due to several factors.

First of all, RS and other micrognathic patients are an inhomogeneous group.[2] Syndromic RS patients tend to be more severely affected than nonsyndromic RS patients. Other diagnoses associated with micrognathia such as Nager, Treacher Collins, and craniofacial microsomia are frequently worse as well. Secondly, there is significant variation in patient population presenting to various institutions. This variation depends on numerous factors. Location of the center is one of the most important. The larger the referral base, the more likely the center is to have exposure to rare conditions. If that center has trained many providers who remain in the area, those providers can manage the more straightforward patients referring on only the most challenging cases. Large metropolitan areas might have several centers competing for patients. One of the more interesting factors is the specialty of the provider. It has been suggested that certain specialties tend to favor one management option over the others. The choice seems to come down to training, experience and comfort level with the various options. That being said, there is some useful information in the literature.

It is reasonable to say there is a consensus in the literature that RS patients should be managed with a spectrum of intervention that is appropriate to severity.[3] Where the controversy begins is after positioning, special feeding techniques, supplemental feeding and temporary airway adjuvants fail.[4] Abel and colleagues[5] recently reported 86.5% of their Robin patients managed successfully with positioning or nasopharyngeal airways. Relatively long term home use of nasopharyngeal airways has been suggested.[6] The surgical interventions of lip-tongue adhesion (LTA), MDO and tracheotomy all have their costs and benefits. The trend is to save tracheotomy for those who fail the first two because once trached these patients tend to not be decannulatable for several years. LTA has waned a little as well, but there are still strong advocates.[7] Cost has recently been looked at as a factor, and tracheotomy loses there because of the long term care needs. The difficulty is knowing which patients will benefit most from each intervention. Recently the GILLS score (gastroesophageal reflux disease, intubation, late airway surgery, low birth weight) has been shown to have predictive value for LTA.[8] Neurologic impairment has been added to this list as well.[9] Additionally, other airway pathology worsens the prognosis.

To summarize, most PRS patients will be successfully managed with nonsupine positioning, special feeding techniques and temporary nasopharyngeal airway support allowing growth and maturation to reduce the problems. Patients with gastroesophageal reflux disease, requiring intubation in the first 24 hours, of low birth weight, or with neurologic or other airway impairment are more likely to need surgical intervention. My first choice is MDO except for the patients with severe neurologic impairment or other airway pathology. They are more likely to be managed with tracheotomy.

What role does DO have in adult orthognathic surgery situations?

SIDMAN

DO for the mandible is almost never indicated in adults as sagittal split osteotomy is the procedure of choice. It is indicated in midface deficiency if there is a need to bring the maxilla forward more than 10 to 12 mm. Single stage movement of this amount will result in some relapse due to the pressure of the soft tissue envelope. In this case, maxillary DO would be indicated even in an adult. Most of the time, two jaw (mandible and maxilla) surgery is needed in these cases.

In summary, only the most severe midface deficiency patients need maxillary distraction, and virtually no adult patients need mandibular distraction.

TATUM

This is an interesting question. The adult orthognathic surgery population is also heterogeneous. There are those patients with lifelong malocclusion and skeletal disharmony who have decided to address the problem for whatever reason in adulthood rather than earlier. These patients typically do not have major skeletal discrepancies (greater than 6–8 mm) and do not require large movements. The main advantages of distraction over conventional orthognathic surgery are the gradual application of soft tissue stretch and the elimination of bone grafts for large moves.[10] Distraction does not generally offer an advantage over traditional orthognathic surgery procedures such as the Le Fort I and the sagittal split ramus osteotomies for these patients. A couple of exceptions are when bone grafts are needed such as for maxillary down grafting or possibly in patients over 40 for whom the risk of bad splits and permanent inferior alveolar nerve injury increases with sagittal split osteotomies. Additionally, those with significant scarring such as cleft patients can benefit.[11] Cleft patients also benefit from gradual movement being less likely to cause velopharyngeal insufficiency than all at once movements.

The occasional patient who makes it to adulthood with large skeletal discrepancies that would involve significant soft tissue stretch and bone grafts to correct would be a good candidate for distraction. The soft tissue stretch is gradual and bone grafts are not needed.

Another situation where distraction might be desirable in the adult patient is in the management of obstructive sleep apnea. These patients may or may not have malocclusion and/or skeletal discrepancy, but either way the goal is typically to expand the upper airway as much as possible. These patients often require movements or one or both jaws of greater than 10 mm. The catch is that the movements of both jaws must be perfectly coordinated to maintain presurgical occlusion or result in a desired occlusal change in coordination with orthodontic therapy. This task is arguably easier when the movements are made all at once and fixated in precise positions. However, finishing orthodontics is frequently necessary to fine tune the occlusion after conventional orthognathic surgery, and it can also assist in achieving good final occlusion after distraction. Finally, in some situations the techniques are being integrated to provide the best of both for the patient.[12,13]

In monobloc and Le Fort III procedures, are internal or external devices preferable?

SIDMAN

We have little experience with this, but when we do need to, we use external devices with concomitant orthodontic devices for guidance of trajectory and occlusion.

TATUM

Both types of devices can achieve good results.[14] Some surgeons have used them together.[15] The exposure and osteotomies are similar. There are numerous differences, advantages and disadvantages. External devices pull the distracted segment forward from multiple attachment points. Internal devices push the segment forward from laterally. The external devices have the obvious burden of the visible bulk and constant presence around the head and face interfering with activity and potentially becoming dislodged. There is a risk of pin perforation of the skull and meningitis or brain damage. They cause additional scalp

scarring often cause some facial scarring depending on distractor attachment points.

The main advantages of an external device are the multivector control over the distracting segment, multiple attachment points in the midface, and the easy removal of the device after the consolidation phase. The multivector control allows for "on the fly" adjustments of distracting segment movement and very precise fine tuning of the occlusion. The multiple attachment points combat the tendency of the central and lateral portions of the midface to distract at different rates due to different resistance to skeletal movement at those locations. Device removal is a brief incisionless procedure involving loosening this screws.

Internal devices avoid the bulky exposed device although the activators must remain exposed typically behind the ears. Once they are secured in place they are unlikely to migrate or become dislodged. The main disadvantages are no vector adjustability and a fairly major procedure to remove the devices. The procedure must be very carefully planned. Once the devices are placed, the final position of the distracted segment is set. The only choice is to continue activation or to stop. Some minor adjustments can be achieved with orthodontic appliances and elastics. Device removal involves completely repeating the initial exposure to place the devices. It can be even more difficult because the distraction places the distal end of the device further away from the initial incision.[16]

What role does DO play in craniofacial microsomia?

SIDMAN

We have gotten away from mandible DO for hemifacial microsomia as we have found that the midpoint of the chin shifts too far to the normal side. We will perform DO after condylar reconstruction if needed to improve the airway enough to allow for tracheostomy decannulation.

TATUM

Severe cases of craniofacial microsomia (hemifacial microsomia) remain one of the greatest challenges in my practice. The significant soft and hard tissue defects as well as the asymmetries can be very difficult to manage. Additionally, the interplay of intervention and growth has made timing of intervention very controversial. Traditional treatment involves coordinated orthodontic measures and surgical intervention. The orthodontics can involve braces and/or functional appliances often timed to take advantage of growth spurts. The surgical procedures involve the addition of bone in the posterior mandible. This might entail replacing the deficient condyle and ramus with a rib graft. Or if the condyle is present, but the ramus is deficient an interposition graft of iliac or calvarium can be placed in an inverted "L" or "C" osteotomy. The child has to obtain sufficient growth to allow for bone graft of adequate size. The growth potential of this graft is difficult to predict also. Occlusal plane leveling Le Fort I osteotomies might be needed as well if the cant is too severe or the midline rotation is too great.

DO allows for earlier intervention than traditional surgery, useful in cases of airway compromise where tracheotomy might be avoided. An infant too young for rib grafting can undergo DO to improve upper airway obstruction due to mandibular deficiency.[17] Frequently in these cases the mandible is deficient on both sides (albeit asymmetrically) and bilateral DO is necessary. The problems are not harming the dentition with the osteotomy or the distractor fixation and, in severe cases, the lack of bone stock for distraction and the resistance of the deficient soft tissue to stretch. In the most severe cases with a complete condyle and ramus defect, a transport disk must be cut from the existing mandible end and distracted posteriorly until it contacts the skull base before any forward motion of the mandible can occur. This distraction vector is usually not linear. It is angulated (multivector) or curvilinear and can be quite complex to plan. The final position of the distracted segment is frequently not what was predicted. Even in less severe cases where the mandible is complete, just small, and elongational DO is employed, the vectors of distraction are difficult to select. Computer planning is helpful in determining the correct osteotomy site and angulation, the type of device, and the orientation of the device.[18] Simultaneous distraction of the maxilla and mandible is becoming a more popular approach to deal with the more severe of the dentofacial asymmetries.[19]

Is endoscopic DO better than open procedures for synostosis management?

SIDMAN

We have not performed endoscopic DO for craniosynostosis, and have only performed open cranial DO for one case of multiple suture synostosis, with a terrific result. We have not yet reported this.

TATUM

This question represents one of the new frontiers in distraction. Distraction has been used for many years for the monobloc advancement procedure which had previously had a very high complication rate related to the wide connection between the sinonasal and intracranial spaces. More recently distraction has been applied to scaphocephaly, plagiocephaly, and brachycephaly. The promise of achieving craniofacial corrections minimally invasively and gradually is attractive. The reduction in blood loss, brain and ocular manipulation and cost is desirable although the second procedure to remove the device(s) is a drawback. The question is are the results similar or better.

In scaphocephaly synostectomy is performed endoscopically, and the cranial length is expected to decrease secondarily due to external molding from sleep position or a helmet.[20] In another method a hand made wire spring is placed across the suture to push it apart. The rapid rate of this movement has led many to claim that it is not true distraction. A distractor typically moves no faster than 3 mm per day. Whether a wire spring or true distractor is used, the skull is actively widened across the opened sagittal suture. The orbits are not involved, and there generally is little asymmetry. This type of procedure seems to work well for scaphocephaly although it is less effective for managing the frontal bossing that is often present. It is as effective for select cases as traditional techniques with the above mentioned advantages.

Brachycephaly presents a challenge to conventional craniofacial surgery. These patients need significant cranial expansion to relieve intracranial constraint causing elevated pressure and contributing to Chiari related problems and venous outflow.[21] The anteroposterior diameter of the skull must be increased against significant soft tissue resistance and the usual supine sleep position pushing the occiput forward. Posterior cranial expansion with distraction as with anterior monobloc distraction offers a significant improvement over traditional techniques. The posterior dissection is safer as osteotomies are performed without bone removal and less dural elevation is required in the area of the large posterior dural sinuses. The soft tissue and sleep position forces are gradually overcome by the devices, and greater overall expansion can be achieved.

Plagiocephaly whether frontal or occipital involves significant asymmetry. The planning and execution of cranial or cranio-orbital distraction to achieve symmetry is difficult. The posterior plagiocephaly from lambdoid synostosis might be improved by distraction without total symmetry being critical. Frontal plagiocephaly from coronal synostosis requires fairly precise positioning of the moved bone segments. Additionally the contralateral compensatory frontal bossing needs to be addressed separately from the retruded side being treated by DO. Achieving fronto-orbital symmetry under these circumstances with DO is challenging. The reports of using DO in these situations mostly cover carefully selected cases suitable for the technique such as very young infants. Additionally, helmets are often required as well.[22]

Trigonocephaly from metopic synostosis has the advantage of symmetry over plagiocephaly, but the concerns are similar. The deformity typically requires differential advancement of the fronto-orbital segments. The lateral aspects require up to 2 cm of advancement whereas there is little or no need for advancement centrally. This is a complex curvilinear movement significantly opening the interfrontal and closing the frontotemporal angles. Distraction does not currently offer an advantage over standard open procedures for this condition either.[23]

Analysis: how has your technique changed or evolved over the past 5 years and what has doing this technique taught you?

SIDMAN

We have now done DO of the mandible on over 100 children, and have reported extensively on this in the literature. There are a number of things we have learned. We will not do this on babies smaller than 2000 g as the mandible is too soft. We leave them intubated until they reach the 2 kg milestone. We have found that children with multiple medical problems, especially significant neurologic issues are the ones most likely to fail DO. Some of these children will still end up with a tracheotomy, and more will end up with a gastrostomy even if the airway is fine.

I am frequently asked about submerged versus external distractors. I have not found external scars to be a major issue in these children who have undergone external DO. The internal devices have two potential problems. The first is getting the vectors off even slightly can result in an open bite that cannot be corrected with the distractors and will require another operation later. This is not an issue with external DO as the open bite can be corrected with the multidirectional devices. The second issue with the internal (submerged) devices is that it requires a second operation to remove them, and I believe this is where the underreported, but not infrequent complication of facial paralysis comes from. With migration of the posterior segment from remodeling of the bone and TM joint, the distractor sits right by the stylomastoid foramen and the main trunk of the facial nerve. Exposure of the distractor plate requires significant retraction of the soft tissues, and potential trauma to the facial nerve. Nonetheless, if a surgeon is getting good results without open bites, or facial nerve paresis problems, then there is certainly no reason not to use submerged distractors.

Taking care to identify the inner angle of the mandible and differentiate this landmark from the condylar notch is critical. Care to make sure that the osteotomies are complete at the time of the surgery is also critical as the pediatric mandible will not fracture from the pressure of the distractors. The surgeon will be fooled by movement of the distractors when all that is really happening is migration of the pins and screws through the bone. This gives the false impression of distraction when in fact no real movement is taking place.

In our program, we have found the collaboration between Otolaryngology and Oral Surgery to be invaluable. Each specialist brings a unique viewpoint to the table, and we both have learned tremendously from each other through years of collaboration. While the Otolaryngologist brings significant soft tissue skills to the patient, the Oral Surgeon brings a unique knowledge of bony manipulation and occlusion into play. Having worked in three different major medical centers in my career, I have found this partnership with Oral Surgery to be easy to establish and maintain. I strongly encourage other members of our specialty to seek out this collaboration for craniofacial reconstructive surgery.

TATUM

Some of the problems I have encountered with DO in the past 5 years can be divided into four phases: planning, osteotomy and placement, activation and consolidation, and removal. In the planning phase potential mistakes include wrong vector, wrong osteotomy or device orientation, wrong device type, incomplete osteotomy or failure of planning model to accurately predict the complex movement of the distracted segment.

In the osteotomy and device placement phase the main problem is failure to accurately follow the plan. Soft tissue damage can occur. Another issue is inadequate bone stock for making the osteotomy and placing device fixation screws far enough away from bone edges and without damaging tooth roots and neurovascular structures.

During activation infection around the device can occur. The activator can spontaneously turn against the distraction direction, the person doing the activation can turn the activator the wrong way. The device can fail either by fracture or malfunction of the distraction mechanism. During activation or consolidation the device can lose fixation and become unstable or become infected. During consolidation mineralization can fail to occur adequately.

During device removal the same problems as with device placement can occur. Additionally, because the DO process involves movement, one end or the other of the device might be significantly further from the incision than when it was placed making removal more difficult.

Numerous technical refinements from the device makers have addressed some of these problems. The devices are being made smaller and stronger. Some have ratcheting mechanisms to prevent backwards movement. The activator tools usually now have direction indicators to reduce wrong direction activation. Screws and footplates have been enhanced to increase fixation stability.

Some of the things I do differently now include more time on family education regarding activation and skin care around the activators. I try to have the activators stick out less by placing them less prominently and adding extenders during the distraction process if the end of the activator gets too close to the skin surface. I tend to use more screws for fixation (4–5 per side), and I try to reduce the number of times I bend the foot plates during contouring to reduce metal fatigue. I use detachable foot plates whenever practical to reduce the difficulty of device removal. I also have increased my consolidation time to three times the distraction time.

By far the biggest change I have made in recent years is to take advantage of the surgical CAD/CAM services now offered by several companies.

The ability to simulate the movement of the distracted segment is a big advantage in planning osteotomy location, device type, placement, and distraction vector(s). The complexity of the geometry and soft tissue interplay are not perfectly modeled by the programs yet so the actual outcomes still differ a little from the planned ones. However, as more outcomes data is collected, the accuracy will improve.

Finally, I have narrowed my indications for DO over the years. There are still areas where distraction is being used for which I have returned to traditional techniques. High grade craniofacial microsomia for example is a condition that I use less distraction and more bone grafting for than I did 5 years ago. The poor bone stock in these patients is the main reason. On the other hand, I use distraction for cranial vault expansion now, and I was not doing that 5 years ago.

What I have learned is that like any other new tool in our armamentarium, DO has been going through its proliferative phase where people were trying it for anything to see how it worked like we are currently doing with robotic surgery. As 14 years of experience has developed, distraction has demonstrated areas of strength and weakness relative to traditional techniques. In situations where there is good starting bone stock, large movements are needed, and there is significant resistance to the movement, distraction is typically superior. For small movements and situations with poor bone stock traditional osteotomies and bone grafting tend to be better.

REFERENCES: TATUM

1. Judge B, Hamlar D, Rimell FL. Mandibular distraction osteogenesis in a neonate. Arch Otolaryngol Head Neck Surg 1999;125(9):1029–32.
2. Breugem CC, Mink van der Molen AB. What is 'Pierre Robin sequence'? J Plast Reconstr Aesthet Surg 2009;62(12):1555–8.
3. Mackay DR. Controversies in the diagnosis and management of the Robin sequence. J Craniofac Surg 2011;22(2):415–20.
4. Bookman LB, Melton KR, Pan BS, et al. Neonates with tongue-based airway obstruction: a systematic review. Otolaryngol Head Neck Surg 2012;146(1): 8–18.
5. Abel F, Bajaj Y, Wyatt M, et al. The successful use of the nasopharyngeal airway in Pierre Robin sequence: an 11-year experience. Arch Dis Child 2012;97(4):331–4.
6. Mondini CC, Marques IL, Fontes CM, et al. Nasopharyngeal intubation in Robin sequence: technique and management. Cleft Palate Craniofac J 2009; 46(3):258–61.
7. Cozzi F, Totonelli G, Frediani S, et al. The effect of glossopexy on weight velocity in infants with Pierre Robin syndrome. J Pediatr Surg 2008;43(2): 296–8.
8. Abramowicz S, Bacic JD, Mulliken JB, et al. Validation of the GILLS score for tongue-lip adhesion in Robin sequence patients. J Craniofac Surg 2012; 23(2):382–6.
9. Tonsager SC, Mader NS, Sidman JD, et al. Determining risk factors for early airway intervention in newborns with micrognathia. Laryngoscope 2012; 122(Suppl 4):S103–4.
10. Bouchard C, Troulis MJ, Kaban LB. Management of obstructive sleep apnea: role of distraction osteogenesis. Oral Maxillofac Surg Clin North Am 2009;21(4):459–75.
11. Cheung LK, Chua HD. Distraction or orthognathic surgery for cleft lip and palate patients: which is better? Ann R Australas Coll Dent Surg 2008;19: 133–5.
12. Resnick CM, Kaban LB, Troulis MJ. Minimally invasive orthognathic surgery. Facial Plast Surg 2009; 25(1):49–62.
13. Schendel SA. Treatment of maxillomandibular deformities with internal curvilinear distraction. Ann Plast Surg 2011;67(6):S1–9.
14. Marchac A, Arnaud E. Cranium and midface distraction osteogenesis: current practices, controversies, and future applications. J Craniofac Surg 2012; 23(1):235–8.
15. Nishimoto S, Oyama T, Tei S, et al. "Bibloc advancement" with a combination of internal and external distracters. J Craniofac Surg 2012;23(5):1444–7.
16. Meling TR, Hogevold HE, Due-Tonnessen BJ, et al. Midface distraction osteogenesis: internal vs. external devices. Int J Oral Maxillofac Surg 2011; 40(2):139–45.
17. Molina F. Mandibular distraction osteogenesis: a clinical experience of the last 17 years. J Craniofac Surg 2009;20(Suppl 2):1794–800.
18. Kim S, Seo YJ, Choi TH, et al. New approach for the surgico-orthodontic treatment of hemifacial microsomia. J Craniofac Surg 2012;23(4):957–63.
19. Ogata H, Sakamoto Y, Sakamoto T, et al. Maxillomandibular tandem osteotomy with distraction osteogenesis for hemifacial microsomia. J Craniofac Surg 2012;23(5):1362–3.
20. Berry-Candelario J, Ridgway EB, Grondin RT, et al. Endoscope-assisted strip craniectomy and

Index

Note: Page numbers of article titles are in **boldface** type.

A

Ablative resurfacing. See *Laser ablative resurfacing.*
Adamson and Kim, on rhinoplasty, alloplastic vs.
  autologous implants for, 39–41
    endonasal approach to, 30
    evolution, observations, and lessons learned,
      47–49
    open vs. closed approach to, 26–27
    reduction, spreader grafts for reduction of
      upper lateral cartilage, 43–44, 49
    tip lobule as divided or preserved in, 31–35
      intraoperative photographs of, 32
      schematic procedural illustrations of, 33
      vertical division of M-arch and, 31–32
Adamson and Warner, on revision rhinoplasty
  alloplasts in, 80–83
    dorsal augmentation in, best substance for
      when cartilage not available, 64–66
      prevention of warping of rib cartilage grafts,
        70
    single most difficult challenge in, 57–58
    spreader grafts for reduction of upper lateral
      cartilage, 75–76
Adamson, Peter A., MD, on revision rhinoplasty. See
  Adamson and Warner.
  on rhinoplasty. See *Adamson and Kim.*
Adipocytes, physiology of, 130
Adult orthognathic surgery, distraction osteogenesis
  role in, 140–141
    Sidman on, 140–141
    Tatum on, 141
Advanced Fitzpatrick skin types, chemical peels in,
  12–13
    Cortez on, 12
    Fedok on, 12
    Mangat on, 12–13
    spot testing with agents for, 11
Aesthetic aspects, of lower lid blepharoplasty, 101,
  112, 116–117
  of midface lift, 120, 132, 135
  of rhinoplasty, 51–52
    revision, 58, 75, 86, 88
    spreader grafts and, reduction, 44, 46, 52
      revision, 75–76, 79
Age/aging, in facial rejuvenation. See *Facial aging.*
Airway adjuvants, for micrognathia, 139–140
Airway compromise, distraction osteogenesis and,
  143

in neonates. See *Micrognathia.*
    distraction osteogenesis for. See *Neonatal
      distraction osteogenesis.*
  with craniofacial microsomia, 142
Alar base, over-resection of, in revision rhinoplasty,
  60–61
  reduction of, in rhinoplasty, 49
Alar cartilage, in rhinoplasty, strength and position of,
  52
    vertical dome division and, 35–37
    vertical lobule division and, 35
Alar crease, in rhinoplasty, 52
Alar deformities, in revision rhinoplasty, as difficult,
  59–62
Alar notching/retraction, in revision rhinoplasty,
  60–61, 63
Alar rim, in rhinoplasty, 52
Alloderm, in rhinoplasty, 41
Allografts, in rhinoplasty, 39. See also *specific graft.*
    advantage of, 40–41
    complications of, 41–42
    evolution of, 50
    sources of, 42
Alloplastic implants. See also *specific implant.*
  in midface lift, 129–130
  in revision rhinoplasty, 80–85
    Adamson and Warner on, 80–83
    Becker on, 83
    for dorsal augmentation, 67, 80, 83–84
    Romo on, 83–85
    Toriumi on, 85
  in rhinoplasty, vs. autologous implants, 39–43, 51
Alloplastic vs. autologous implants, for rhinoplasty,
  39–43
    Adamson and Kim on, 39–41
    Constantinides on, 41–42, 51
    Pearlman on, 42–43
Antibiotics, pre-peel use of, 17
Antivirals, pre-peel use of, 17
Antunes, Marcelo B., MD, on midface lift. See *Quatela
  and Antunes.*
Arch symmetry, in rhinoplasty, tip lobule division vs.
  preservation and, 38
    vertical dome division and, 35–37
    vertical lobule division and, 33–34
Arcus marginalis, in lower lid blepharoplasty,
  104–105, 114
  in midface lift, 125–126, 129–130

Moving?

Make sure your subscription moves with you!

To notify us of your new address, find your **Clinics Account Number** (located on your mailing label above your name), and contact customer service at:

Email: journalscustomerservice-usa@elsevier.com

800-654-2452 (subscribers in the U.S. & Canada)
314-447-8871 (subscribers outside of the U.S. & Canada)

Fax number: 314-447-8029

Elsevier Health Sciences Division
Subscription Customer Service
3251 Riverport Lane
Maryland Heights, MO 63043

*To ensure uninterrupted delivery of your subscription, please notify us at least 4 weeks in advance of move.

Printed and bound by CPI Group (UK) Ltd, Croydon, CR0 4YY

03/10/2024

01040356-0005